DEJA REVIEW™

USMLE Step 2 CK

D1016842

DEJA REVIEW™
USMLE Step 2 CK

Second Edition

John H. Naheedy, MD
Fellow, Pediatric Radiology
Department of Radiology
Children's Hospital Boston
Harvard Medical School
Boston, Massachusetts

Daniel A. Orringer, MD
Chief Resident
Department of Neurosurgery
University of Michigan Medical School
Ann Arbor, Michigan

Khashayar Mohebali, MD
Chief Resident, Clinical Instructor
Division of Plastic and Reconstructive Surgery
Department of Surgery
University of California, San Francisco
San Francisco, California

Peter F. Aziz, MD
Fellow-Pediatric Cardiology
Department of Pediatrics
Children's Hospital of Philadelphia
Philadelphia, Pennsylvania

Susie Lim, MD
Clinical Instructor
Obstetrics and Gynecology
Kaiser Permanente Northwest
Portland, Oregon

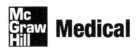

New York   Chicago   San Francisco   Lisbon   London   Madrid   Mexico City
Milan   New Delhi   San Juan   Seoul   Singapore   Sydney   Toronto

The McGraw·Hill Companies

Déjà Review™ USMLE Step 2 CK, Second Edition

1 2 3 4 5 6 7 8 9 0   DOC/DOC   14 13 12 11 10

ISBN 978-0-07-162716-0
MHID 0-07-162716-2

This book was set in Palatino by Glyph International.

The editors were Kirsten Funk and Peter J. Boyle.

The production supervisor was Catherine H. Saggese.

Project management was provided by Harleen Chopra, Glyph International.

RR Donnelley was printer and binder.

This book is printed on acid-free paper.

Cataloging-in-publication data is on file for this book at the Library of Congress.

McGraw-Hill books are available at special quantity discounts to use as premiums and sales promotions, or for use in corporate training programs. To contact a representative please e-mail us at bulksales@mcgraw-hill.com.

To my family and friends,
for their love and encouragement;
and to my parents,
for being an example of everything I want to be.
—John

To Megan, the true author in the family.
—Dan

To my parents for dedicating and sacrificing their lives
to make mine better
and to my friends
for their invaluable loyalty.
—Khashi

To my family,
for teaching me that the love of medicine
can be genetically inherited;
and to the bunker, the sand trap of my closest friends,
thanks for the inspiration.
—Pete

To Michael, Oliver and Soë
—Susie

Contents

Contributors

Karla Fredricks, MD
Resident
Department of Pediatrics
Children's Hospital of Philadelphia
Philadelphia, Pennsylvania
Chapter: Pediatrics

Emily Y. Fukuchi, MD
Resident
Department of Obstetrics and Gynecology
University of California, San Francisco
San Francisco, California
Chapters: Internal Medicine, Surgery

Karen A. Kinnaman, MD
University of Michigan Medical School
Ann Arbor, Michigan
Class of 2009
Chapter: Emergency Medicine

Vijay Pottathil, MD
Resident
Department of Internal Medicine
University of Iowa
Iowa City, Iowa
Chapter: Internal Medicine

Jayson Sack, MD
Resident
Department of Neurosurgery
University of South Florida
Tampa, Florida
Chapters: Neurology, Psychiatry

Miguel Trujillo, MD
Resident
Department of Obstetrics and Gynecology
Oregon Health and Science University
Portland, Oregon
Chapter: Obstetrics and Gynecology

Reviewers

Jessica Bury, MPH
Medical Student
Mayo Clinical College of Medicine
Class of 2010

Tina Nguyen, MD
Resident, Emergency Medicine
Harbor UCLA Medical Center
University of California Los Angeles
SUNY Upstate Medical University
Class of 2008

Preface

Déjà Review™ USMLE Step 2 CK has been scrutinized and edited to produce a second edition that is even higher yield and easier to use than the first. Outstanding medical students, who have recently taken Step 2, revised the original text to ensure the material covered herein is complete and current. The authors, now with a combined 30 years of experience in the medical field, have also edited the manuscript to emphasize the clinical relevance of the core concepts covered in Step 2. We are confident that our efforts have produced one of the most useful guides for Step 2 review available today.

Step 2 of the United States Medical Licensing Examination (USMLE) tests the senior medical student's ability to apply the basic principles of clinical medicine. However, before you can apply those principles, you must be able to rapidly recall a core body of essential facts. This is why the Déjà Review series is the most efficient, well-organized, portable, and above all, high-yield resource to prepare students for the USMLE. As recent graduates who have taken Step 2, we are confident that we have compiled a novel review guide that promotes rapid recall of all of the essential facts necessary for success on this examination. We also realize that a solid foundation in these principles will allow you to make a smooth transition into your residency.

ORGANIZATION

All concepts are presented in a question and answer format that covers the key facts on hundreds of common and uncommon diseases. The material is divided into chapters covering the six major divisions of clinical medicine: internal medicine, surgery, neuroscience, psychiatry, OB/GYN, and pediatrics. We have also included a brief emergency medicine chapter that addresses topics not covered under emergent conditions in each of the other chapters.

This question and answer format has several important advantages:
- It provides a rapid, straightforward way for you to assess your strengths and weaknesses.
- It allows you to efficiently review and commit to memory a large body of information.
- It will prepare you for getting "pimped" by residents and attendings on the wards.
- It offers you a break from tedious, convoluted multiple-choice questions.
- The clinical vignettes will expose you to the prototypic presentation of diseases classically tested on the USMLE Step 2.
- It serves as a quick, last-minute review of high-yield facts.

The compact, condensed design of the book is conducive to studying on the go, especially during any downtime on the wards.

HOW TO USE THIS BOOK

Remember, this text is not intended to replace textbooks, course packs, or lectures. It is, however, intended to serve as a supplement to your studies during the third and fourth years of medical school. This text has been sampled and refined by a number of medical students who found it to be an essential part of their preparation for the USMLE shelf examinations, in addition to Step 2 itself. We recommend having the text spiral bound to make it more portable and easier to use. Begin using this book early in your third year by carrying it with you during your clinical clerkships. You may cover up the answers with the included bookmark and quiz yourself or even your classmates. For a greater challenge, try covering up the questions!

However you choose to study, we hope you find this resource helpful during your preparation for the USMLE Step 2 and throughout your clinical rotations. Best of luck!

John H. Naheedy, MD
Daniel A. Orringer, MD
Khashayar Mohebali, MD
Peter F. Aziz, MD
Susie Lim, MD

Acknowledgments

The authors would like to thank the following individuals for their invaluable contributions to this text and their efforts in making this a useful resource for students:

Deborah A. Bartholomew, MD
Clinical Associate Professor
Department of Obstetrics and Gynecology
Ohio State University Medical Center
Columbus, Ohio

Peter Muscarella II, MD
Assistant Professor, Clinical
Department of Surgery
Ohio State University Medical Center
Columbus, Ohio

Emile El-Shammaa, MD
Assistant Professor, Clinical
Department of Emergency Medicine
Department of Pediatrics
Columbia, Ohio
Ohio State University Medical Center
Columbus, Ohio

The authors would like to recognize the faculty and staff at the Ohio State University College of Medicine for their endless commitment to education. Without the wisdom and encouragement of mentors like the late John M. Stang, MD, this project would not have been possible. We would also like to thank the students who used this text in preparation for their boards and provided feedback essential to optimizing this text. Finally, special thanks to our managing editor Kirsten Funk for her dedication and patience.

CHAPTER 1

Internal Medicine

CARDIOLOGY

Hypertension

What percentage of hypertensive patients have essential hypertension (HTN)?	90%-95%

Name the cause of secondary (2°) HTN in the following clinical scenarios:

HTN upper extremities; decreased or normal blood pressure (BP) in lower extremities	Coarctation of the aorta
HTN accompanied by proteinuria in a nondiabetic patient	Glomerular disease
HTN in a patient with a history of (h/o) renal and hepatic cysts	Polycystic kidney disease
Sudden worsening of HTN in an elderly male with coronary artery disease (CAD) and peripheral vascular disease (PVD)	Renal artery stenosis
Episodic HTN, weight loss, headache, and diaphoresis	Pheochromocytoma
Elevated systolic HTN without diastolic HTN	Hyperthyroidism
40-year-old (y/o) female with a h/o 20 years of oral contraceptive pills (OCP) use	Drug-induced (OCP) HTN
HTN in a patient with hypokalemic metabolic alkalosis	Conn syndrome/hyperaldosteronism
HTN in an overweight patient with buffalo hump, moon facies, hirsutism, and abdominal striae	Cushing syndrome

What is the difference between hypertensive urgency and hypertensive emergency?	In hypertensive urgency there are no signs of end-organ damage due to HTN. In hypertensive emergency there are signs of organ damage (papilledema, renal failure, heart failure, stroke).
What is the treatment of hypertensive urgency?	Oral BP medication (labetalol, captopril, clonidine)
What are the three preferred agents for the treatment of hypertensive emergency?	1. IV nitroprusside 2. Nitroglycerine 3. Hydralazine
What is the preferred treatment for hypertension in pregnancy?	Hydralazine and clonidine or methyldopa

For each of the following conditions, select the best antihypertensive agent(s):

No comorbidities	Diuretics or β-blockers
Isolated systolic HTN	Thiazide diuretics
Angina pectoris	β-Blockers, calcium channel blockers
Diabetes	Angiotensin-converting enzyme inhibitors (ACEi) or angiotensin receptor blocker (ARB), β-blockers
Hyperlipidemia	ACEi, calcium channel blockers
Congestive heart failure (CHF)	Diuretics, ACEi
H/o myocardial infarction (MI)	β-blockers, ACEi
Chronic renal failure	Diuretics, calcium channel blockers
Asthma, chronic obstructive pulmonary disease (COPD)	Diuretics, calcium channel blockers
Benign prostatic hyperplasia (BPH)	α_1-selective antagonist (terazosin)
Pheochromocytoma	Phenoxybenzamine ($\alpha_1\alpha_2$-antagonist), phentolamine (α_1-blocker)
Hypertrophic obstructive cardiomyopathy	β-blockers
Hyperthyroidism	β-blockers
Anxiety	β-blockers
Supraventricular tachycardia (SVT)	β-blockers
Migraine headaches	β-blockers, calcium channel blockers
Moderate bradycardia	β-blockers with intrinsic sympathomimetic activity: pindolol and acebutolol
Osteoporosis	Thiazide diuretics (reabsorbs Ca^{2+})

For each of the following conditions, list the antihypertensive agent(s) that should be used with caution:

CHF	Verapamil, α-blockers
Asthma, COPD	β-blockers
Diabetes	β-blockers, thiazides
Renal artery stenosis, renal failure	ACE inhibitors

Hypercholesterolemia

What genetic disease should be suspected in a patient with xanthomas, xanthelasmas, and lipemia retinalis?

Familial hypercholesterolemia

State the recommended therapeutic intervention or further workup (w/u) for patients with the following lipid values:

Total cholesterol <200	Retest in 5 years
Total cholesterol >200	Treat based on lipid fractions
Low-density lipoprotein (LDL) >190	Begin lipid-lowering therapy (goal <160)
LDL >160 in a patient with two or more coronary risk factors	Begin lipid-lowering therapy (goal <130)
LDL >130 in a patient with CAD or diabetes mellitus (DM)	Begin lipid-lowering therapy (goal <100)
LDL >100 in a patient with a previous MI	Begin lipid-lowering therapy
Triglycerides (TGs) >200	Begin TG-lowering therapy

For each of the following drugs, provide: (1) the mechanism of action (MOA), (2) indication(s) (IND), and (3) significant side effects and unique toxicity (TOX) (if any):

Cholestyramine

MOA: bile-acid–binding resin

IND: adjuvant therapy for patients with familial hypercholesterolemia

TOX: constipation, gastrointestinal (GI) discomfort, may interfere with intestinal absorption of other drugs

Statins	**MOA:** hydroxymethylglutaryl (HMG) coenzyme A (CoA) reductase inhibitors
	IND: hypercholesterolemia
	TOX: hepatotoxicity, rhabdomyolysis
Niacin	**MOA:** reduces release of very low-density lipoprotein (VLDL) from liver into circulation
	IND: hypercholesterolemia: to ↑ high-density lipoprotein (HDL) and ↓ LDL
	TOX: flushing, pruritus (both reversible with aspirin), and hepatotoxicity
Gemfibrozil, clofibrate	**MOA:** stimulates lipoprotein lipase
	IND: hypercholesterolemia: to ↓↓ TGs
	TOX: myositis, hepatotoxicity

Coronary Artery Disease

Which are the six coronary risk factors?	**CAD HDL**
	1. Cigarettes
	2. Age (males >45 and females >55 are at increased risk) and sex (males > females)
	3. Diabetes mellitus (greatest risk factor)
	4. HTN
	5. Death from MI in family history (FH) (males <55 y/o, females <60 y/o)
	6. ↑ LDL, low HDL (<35)
What is the common presentation of a patient with symptomatic CAD?	Angina pectoris ± radiation to jaw, left shoulder, or arm; exacerbated by exertion, relieved by rest, and nitroglycerin
Which groups of patients commonly do *not* exhibit classic anginal symptoms in the setting of myocardial ischemia?	Elderly, women, and diabetics (due to diabetic neuropathy, heart transplant patients)
Which type of angina is characterized by chest pain and dyspnea at rest?	Unstable angina
What are the classic ECG findings during an anginal episode?	>1-mm ST-segment depression and T-wave inversion
What diagnostic tests are often used to screen for CAD?	Exercise or pharmacologic stress test or imaging

Which patients should undergo exercise ECG w/ myocardial imaging + stress echo in the workup of CAD?

Patients with Wolf-Parkinson-White syndrome, >1-mm ST depression on resting ECG; hx of percutaneous transluminal coronary angioplasty (PTCA), on Digoxin, or those with left ventricular hypertrophy (LVH)

Who gets pharmacologic stress test?

Patients with electronically paced ventricular rhythm and left bundle branch block (LBBB)

What is the gold standard for the diagnosis of CAD?

Coronary arteriography

Name six lifestyle changes that should be suggested to all patients with HTN:

1. Weight loss
2. Sodium restriction
3. Physical exercise
4. Smoking cessation
5. Alcohol cessation
6. Stress reduction

What medications should be given to a patient with acute onset of angina?

Sublingual nitroglycerin

What medications should be given as prophylaxis for angina and MI?

Long-acting nitrates, β-blockers, ASA, statin (and ACEI in patients with h/o MI)

What are the key steps in the medical management of a patient with unstable angina?

Start IV, administer O_2, start heparin, ASA, β-blocker, nitroglycerin, morphine

Describe how nitrates reduce angina:

1. Venodilation causes venous pooling →↓ preload →↓ myocardial O_2 consumption
2. Coronary vasodilation →↑ O_2 delivery to the myocardium

What is the most common side effect of nitrates?

Headache

Describe how each of the following drugs reduces angina:

    β-Blockers

↓ Myocardial O_2 use, ↓ afterload, ↑ coronary filling during diastole

    Nifedipine

Coronary arteriolar vasodilation

    Verapamil

Slows cardiac conduction

What is the antianginal drug of choice for prinzmetal angina?

Diltiazem

Which antianginal drug must be used with caution in patients with asthma and COPD?	β-blockers
What intervention is reserved for patients whose angina cannot be controlled medically?	Percutaneous transluminal coronary angioplasty (PTCA)
What are the indications for coronary artery bypass grafting?	Angina refractory to medical therapy, severe left main disease, and triple vessel coronary disease (or double vessel disease in a diabetic)

Myocardial Infarction

What is the common presentation of MI?	Crushing retrosternal chest pressure occurring at rest and radiating to left arm, neck, or jaw; diaphoresis; nausea/vomiting; dyspnea; and anxiety
What is a common physical examination finding during an MI?	S4 gallop
Which are the six life-threatening causes of chest pain that must be ruled out in all patients?	1. MI 2. Aortic dissection 3. Pulmonary embolism (PE) 4. Pneumothorax (PTX) 5. Esophageal rupture 6. Cardiac tamponade
What are the key steps in the initial management of a patient with suspected MI?	Assess vital signs, administer O_2, start IV, place on cardiac monitor, and obtain ECG; administer ASA, heparin, nitrates, β-blockers, morphine, clopidogrel
What are the classic ECG abnormalities in an acute MI?	ST elevation and Q waves
Which ECG finding is very sensitive and specific for right ventricular infarction?	ST elevation of 1 mm in right-sided lead V4
Which coronary artery is likely to be occluded in a patient with the following ECG abnormalities?	
Large R and ST-segment depression in V1, V2	Right coronary (posterior infarction)
Q waves and ST-segment elevation in leads V1-V4	Left anterior descending (anterior infarction)

Q wave in leads I, aVL, V5, V6	Circumflex (lateral infarction)
Q waves and ST elevation in leads II, III, aVF	Right coronary (inferior infarction)
Which serologic markers are typically used to diagnose and follow an MI?	Troponin I and CK-MB
What medication is reserved for patients with MI suffering from angina that is refractory to conventional medical management?	Thrombolytics including tissue plasminogen activator or streptokinase
What intervention is indicated in patients during an MI who fail or cannot tolerate thrombolytic therapy?	PTCA
What are the clinical manifestations of right ventricular MI?	ECG inf. changes, hypotension, clear lungs, jugular venous distension (JVD), right ventricular lift, tricuspid valve regurgitation
Which medical therapy should be avoided in a patient with a right ventricular infarction?	Nitroglycerin (initial therapy should involve IV fluids to ↑ preload)
What long-term medications have been shown to improve mortality in patients with MI?	ASA and β-blockers (acutely); ACEI, statins, and clopidogrel (long term)

Arrhythmias

Name the arrhythmia associated with the following clinical features:	
PR interval >0.2 s, often due to increased vagal tone	Primary (1°) heart block
PR interval gradually increases to the point at which a QRS complex is dropped (P wave is not conducted).	2° Mobitz type I heart block (Wenkebach)
PR interval >0.2 s with occasional dropping of the QRS complex at a fixed interval (ie, 2:1 or 3:1)	2° Mobitz type II heart block
Irregularly irregular pulses and QRS complexes	Atrial fibrillation
Type of heart block that commonly arises as a side effect of medication including β-blockers, digoxin, and calcium channel blockers	2° Mobitz type II heart block

Sawtooth appearance of P waves	Atrial flutter
Usually caused by conduction block within the bundle of His	2° Mobitz type II heart block
Complete dissociation between P waves and QRS complexes	3° or complete heart block
Three or more P-wave morphologies	Multifocal atrial tachycardia if HR >100, wandering pacemaker if HR <100
Associated with cannon A waves in jugular veins and widened pulse pressure	3° heart block
Irregularly irregular pulses and QRS complexes	Atrial fibrillation
Commonly caused by reentry	Paroxsymal SVT
Associated with COPD	Atrial fibrillation, atrial flutter, multifocal atrial tachycardia
Treatment commonly includes anticoagulation, rate control, and/or cardioversion.	Atrial fibrillation
Wide QRS complexes not preceded by a P wave	Premature ventricular contraction (PVC)
Normal QRS morphology with a rate of 150-200 beats/min	Paroxsymal SVT
Pharmocologic treatment includes amiodarone, lidocaine, and procainamide.	Ventricular tachycardia
May be treated with carotid massage or Valsalva maneuver	Paroxsymal SVT
Common cause of palpitation caused by ectopic beats arising from multiple Ventricular foci	PVC
Ventricular arrhythmia commonly caused by myocardial ischemia that may lead to hemodynamic instability	Ventricular tachycardia
First-line therapy is defibrillation; second-line therapy is epinephrine or vasopressin.	Ventricular fibrillation and pulseless ventricular tachycardia
Polymorphic wide complex tachycardia associated with prolonged QT interval	Torsade de pointes
Treated identical to ventricular fibrillation if there is no pulse	Ventricular tachycardia

Tachyarrhythmia treated with adenosine, verapamil, cardioversion, or radiofrequency ablation	Paroxsymal SVT
Narrow complex tachycardia in which P waves follow QRS	Junctional tachycardia or Wolff-Parkinson-White
Treatment with pacemaker is necessary.	Symptomatic 2° Mobitz type II heart block, 3° heart block, and sinus node dysfunction

What is the most common cause of atrial fibrillation?	HTN
What are some other important causes of atrial fibrillation?	**PIRATES** **P**ulmonary disease **I**schemia of myocardium **R**heumatic heart disease **A**nemia or atrial myxoma **T**hyrotoxicosis **E**thanol **S**epsis
What are the two main components in the treatment of atrial fibrilation?	Rate control and long-term anticoagulation (ie, metoprolol and warfarin)
What criteria are used to determine whether warfarin or aspirin is started in the treatment of atrial fibrillation?	CHADS2 score: 1 point for CHF, hypertension, age >75, DM, 2 points for stroke or transient ischemic attack (TIA). Score ≥3 receives warfarin.
Name three clinical scenarios in which atropine is indicated for treatment of a bradyarrhythmia:	1. Bradycardia causing hemodynamic instability 2. Syncope 3. CHF

Congestive Heart Failure

Name six common symptoms of CHF:	1. Dyspnea; exertional initially but occurs at rest as disease progresses 2. Orthopnea 3. Paroxysmal nocturnal dyspnea 4. Cough and wheezing 5. Weight gain due to peripheral edema 6. Worsening fatigue
Name four common signs of left-sided CHF:	1. S3 gallop 2. Inspiratory crackles or rales 3. Laterally displaced point of maximal impulse (due to cardiomegaly) 4. Ventricular heave

Name five common signs of right-sided CHF.	1. Dependent edema 2. Jugular venous distention (JVD) 3. Hepatojugular reflux and ascites 4. Atrial fibrillation 5. Cyanosis
What is the pathophysiologic basis of systolic dysfunction?	Decreased contractility
What are the two common causes of systolic dysfunction?	1. Ischemic cardiomyopathy 2. Ischemic myocarditis
What is the pathophysiologic basis of diastolic dysfunction?	Decreased ventricular compliance
What are the four common causes of diastolic dysfunction?	1. HTN 2. Ischemic cardiomyopathy 3. Hypertrophic cardiomyopathy 4. Systemic disorders (ie, amyloidosis, hemochromatosis)
Name four common chest x-ray (CXR) abnormalities in CHF:	1. Cardiomegaly 2. Cephalization of pulmonary vessels ($\uparrow$ vascularity in lung fields) 3. Kerley B lines (indicating pleural fluid in fissures) 4. Pleural effusions
Name two common echocardiographic abnormalities in CHF:	1. Decreased ejection fraction 2. Cardiomegaly

Name the CHF drug associated with each of the following statements:

Shown to decrease mortality in CHF	ACE inhibitors, β-blockers, and spironolactone ($\downarrow$ mortality in class IV CHF)
Used acutely for worsening dyspnea and fluid retention	Loop diuretics
Reduce afterload by causing vasodilation of both arteries and veins	ACE inhibitors
Reduce symptoms of CHF by improving contractility	Digitalis
Vasodilators used in patients refractory to ACE inhibitors	Hydralazine and isosorbide dinitrate
May cause arrhythmias, yellow-tinted vision, anorexia, and nausea	Digitalis
Intravenous positive inotropic agents	Dopamine, dobutamine, and nesiritide

Valvular Heart Disease

Name the valvular defect associated
with each of the following
murmurs:

Harsh midsystolic murmur in the
right second intercostal space at the
right sternal border, radiating into
the neck and apex

Aortic stenosis

Blowing, high-pitched diastolic
murmur at left two to fourth
interspaces radiating to apex

Aortic regurgitation

Blowing holosystolic murmur at
apex radiating into left axilla with
increased apical impulse

Mitral regurgitation

Low-pitched diastolic murmur at the
apex that gets louder prior to S1; an
opening snap is often present just
after S2

Mitral stenosis

Soft, late systolic murmur at left
sternal border or apex, accompanied
by midsystolic click

Mitral valve prolapse

Harsh midsystolic murmur in the
left second intercostal space at the
left sternal border

Pulmonic stenosis

Blowing holosystolic murmur at
lower left sternal border radiating
to right of sternum; may increase
with inspiration

Tricuspid regurgitation

Harsh holosystolic murmur at lower
left sternal border, accompanied by
thrill

Ventricular septal defect

Harsh midsystolic murmur in the
third and fourth left interspaces
radiating down left sternal border;
S4 and biphasic apical impulse
often present

Hypertrophic cardiomyopathy

Note: the valvular diseases in the
previous answers are in the order
of incidence.

Name the valvular defect associated
with the following features:

Can be caused by papillary muscle
rupture 2° to MI

Mitral regurgitation

May cause left atrial enlargement,
atrial fibrillation, and pulmonary
edema

Mitral stenosis and mitral regurgitation

Presents with triad of angina, syncope, and exertional dyspnea; boot-shaped heart on CXR	Aortic stenosis
May be precipitated by infective endocarditis, aortic aneurysmal dilation, and connective tissue disorders	Aortic insufficiency
Atrioventricular block	Mitral regurgitation
Calcific degeneration of a congenital bicuspid valve	Aortic stenosis
Increased pulse pressure	Aortic insufficiency

Cardiomyopathies

What are the most common etiologies of dilated cardiomyopathy?	ABCD Alcohol abuse Beriberi Coxsackie B myocarditis, cocaine, Chagas disease Doxorubicin toxicity (also pregnancy)
Name the type of cardiomyopathy associated with the following clinical features:	
Asymmetric septal hypertrophy, banana-shaped left ventricle (LV); LV outflow obstruction	Hypertrophic
May be caused by sarcoidosis, amyloidosis, scleroderma, hereditary hemochromatosis, endocardial fibroelastosis, radiation-induced fibrosis	Restrictive
Causes sudden death in young, otherwise healthy athletes	Hypertrophic
Four-chamber hypertrophy and dilation accompanied by systolic dysfunction	Dilated
Cardiomyopathy most commonly caused by endomyocardial fibrosis	Restrictive
Most common type of cardiomyopathy, commonly inherited in autosomal-dominant (AD) fashion	Hypertrophic
ACEi have been demonstrated to decrease mortality	Dilated

Symptoms relieved by squatting (↑ preload)	Hypertrophic
Impaired left ventricular diastolic filling; may mimic constrictive pericarditis	Restrictive
Examination reveals cardiomegaly, mitral regurgitation, and S3; balloon-shaped heart on CXR	Dilated
Mitral regurgitation, sustained apical impulse, S4, and systolic ejection murmur; boot-shaped heart on CXR	Hypertrophic
β-Blockers and calcium channel blockers provide symptomatic relief	Hypertrophic

Pericardial Disease

What is the common presentation of pericarditis?	Pleuritic retrosternal chest pain (↑ when supine, ↓ when sitting up and leaning forward), dyspnea, cough, and fever
What are the most common etiologies of serous pericarditis?	Uremia, systemic lupus erythematosus (SLE), rheumatic fever, coxsackie viral infection
What are the most common etiologies of fibrinous pericarditis?	Uremia, SLE, rheumatic fever, coxsackie viral infection, MI
What are the most common etiologies of hemorrhagic pericarditis?	Trauma, malignancy, tuberculosis
What is a typical examination finding in pericarditis?	Pericardial friction rub
What are the classic ECG findings in pericarditis?	Diffuse ST elevation
What life-threatening complication of pericarditis causes distant heart sounds, JVD, hypotension, pulsus paradoxus, and elevated central venous pressure (CVP) on inspiration?	Cardiac tamponade (Beck's triad = JVD, hypotension, muffled heart sounds)
What is the definitive treatment for acute decompensation in a patient with cardiac tamponade?	Pericardiocentesis
Which 2° intervention may be helpful in the management of a patient with cardiac tamponade?	Intravascular volume expansion

Endocarditis

What are the three major categories of endocarditis?	1. Infective 2. Nonbacterial thrombotic or marantic 3. Libman-Sacks endocarditis
What is the common presentation of infective endocarditis (IE)?	Fever (high in acute endocarditis, low-grade in subacute endocarditis), constitutional symptoms, and dyspnea
What are the clinical signs of IE?	**"JR NO FAME"** Janeway lesions Roth's spots Nail bed hemorrhages Osler's nodes Fever Anemia Murmur Emboli
What criteria are typically used for diagnosing IE?	The Duke criteria
What are the two major Duke criteria?	1. Two consecutive blood cultures (12 h apart) positive for IE-causing organism 2. Echocardiogram demonstrating valvular vegetation, ring abscess, or other evidence of endocardial infection *or* new valve murmur
What are the five minor Duke criteria?	1. Cardiac predisposition including valvular abnormality, congenital heart disease, or hypertrophic cardiomyopathy Risk of bacteremia: DM, indwelling catheter, intravenous drug abuse (IVDA), hemodialysis 2. Fever >38°C (100.4°F) 3. Vascular phenomena: signs of embolic disease including septic pulmonary emboli, mycotic cerebral abscesses, Janeway lesions 4. Immunologic phenomena including Roth spots or Osler nodes 5. Single positive blood culture
How do you make a definitive diagnosis of infective endocarditis?	2 major; 1 major + 3 minor, or 5 minor criteria

What is the most common valve affected by IE? — Mitral valve

What is the most common valve affected by IE in IV drug users? — Tricuspid valve

Name the type of endocarditis described in each of the following clinical scenarios:

25-y/o IV drug user with rapid onset of high fever, rigors, malaise with tricuspid regurgitation — Acute IE

60-y/o female with mitral valve prolapse who has recently undergone dental extraction presenting with low-grade fever and flu-like symptoms — Subacute IE

65-y/o male with metastatic colon cancer and a new murmur consistent with mitral regurgitation — Nonbacterial thrombotic endocarditis

30-y/o female with SLE — Libman-Sacks endocarditis

Which organism most often causes *acute* IE? — *Staphylococcus aureus*

Which organism most often causes *subacute* IE? — *Streptococcus viridans*

Which organisms can cause endocarditis but are not typically isolated by conventional bacterial culture? — **HACEK** organisms (*Haemophilus parainfluenzae, Actinobacillus, Cardiobacterium, Eikenella, Kingella*)

What are some sequelae of bacterial endocarditis? — Valvular injury, renal injury (glomerulonephritis [GN]), septic emboli to brain/lungs/kidneys causing infarction or abscess

What is the most common cause of myocarditis worldwide? — *Trypanosoma cruzii* (Chagas disease)

What is the empiric treatment for a patient with suspected endocarditis (before an organism is isolated in blood cultures)? — An antistaphylococcal β-lactam antibiotic and an aminoglycoside

What is the suggested regimen of antibiotic prophylaxis for patients at increased risk of endocarditis? — Two grams of amoxicillin prior to dental procedures

Which patients should receive endocarditis prophylaxis?	Patients with prosthetic heart valves, previous bacterial endocarditis, high-risk patients (ie, complex cyanotic heart disease), and moderate-risk patients (ie, hypertrophic cardiomyopathy, MVP with regurgitation and/or thickened leaflets, repaired intracardiac defects in past 6 months)

Rheumatic Heart Disease

What type of infection causes rheumatic fever?	Group A streptococcal pharyngitis
How does streptococcal pharyngitis cause rheumatic heart disease?	Antistreptococcal antibodies cross-react with a cardiac antigen.
What serologic test is elevated in rheumatic heart disease?	Antistreptolysin antibodies (ASO), DNAse B
Name the five major Jones criteria for rheumatic heart disease:	"J♥NES" 1. Joints (migratory polyarthritis) 2. ♥: pancarditis 3. N: subcutaneous nodules 4. Erythema marginatum 5. Sydenham chorea
Name three minor Jones criteria for rheumatic heart disease:	1. Fever 2. Arthralgia 3. Leukocytosis
What is the most commonly observed valvular deformity in rheumatic heart disease?	Mitral stenosis
What treatment for streptococcal pharyngitis can prevent rheumatic heart disease?	Penicillin
What is the critical determinant of morbidity in acute rheumatic fever?	Degree of mitral and aortic valve stenosis/regurgitation

Aortic Dissection

What is the typical presentation of an aortic dissection?	Sudden onset of severe, tearing substernal pain radiating to the interscapular region of the back

Which physical examination findings are characteristic of an aortic dissection?

Unequal BP in the extremities, new murmur consistent with aortic regurgitation

What finding on CXR suggests an aortic dissection?

Widened mediastinum

Which coronary artery is most commonly affected by aortic dissection and what are the associated ECG findings?

Right coronary artery. Inferior MI = ST elevation II, III, aVF

What is the gold standard for the diagnosis of aortic dissection?

Angiography (CT with contrast, transesophageal echocardiography, and MRI also have diagnostic use and are less invasive)

What medication is preferred for lowering BP in a patient with an aortic dissection?

Sodium nitroprusside and β-blockers

What is the definitive therapy for an aortic dissection?

Surgical repair

Peripheral Vascular Disease

What are the risk factors for peripheral vascular disease (PVD)?

Similar to coronary risk factors; though diabetes is #1

Name the PVD associated with the following features:

Focal neurologic findings

Cerebrovascular disease

Abdominal pain out of proportion to examination

Mesenteric ischemia

Intermittent claudication

Chronic arterial occlusive disease

Pain in buttocks and thighs with walking

Aortoiliac occlusive disease

Pain in calves with walking

Femoral-popliteal occlusive disease

Abdominal angina

Chronic mesenteric arterial occlusive disease

What noninvasive study is used to diagnose arterial occlusion?

Doppler ultrasound

What is the gold standard for the diagnosis of arterial occlusion?

Angiography

What is the source of most emboli causing acute arterial occlusion?	Cardiac mural thrombus (commonly in patients with atrial fibrillation)
What is the treatment of an acute arterial occlusion?	Surgical or percutaneous thrombectomy or medical thrombolysis
What type of therapy must be administered to all patients with a h/o acute arterial occlusion?	Warfarin

Make the Diagnosis

56-y/o female presents with dyspnea on exertion (DOE); PE (physical examination): loud S1, delayed P2, early diastolic sound, and a diastolic rumble; transesophageal echocardiogram: mobile, pedunculated left atrial mass

Atrial myxoma

60-y/o presents with chest pain relieved by sitting up and leaning forward; PE: pericardial friction rub; ECG: diffuse ST-segment elevation; echocardiogram: pericardial effusion with thickening of the pericardium

Acute pericarditis

65-y/o male presents with 1-week h/o fever and DOE and orthopnea; PE: new blowing holosystolic murmur at apex radiating into left axilla; blood cultures ⊕ for viridans streptococci; echo: oscillating mass attached to mitral valve

Acute IE

60-y/o presents with dyspnea and palpitations; PE: 20 mm Hg decline in systolic BP with inspiration (pulsus paradoxus), ↓ BP, JVD, diminished S1 and S2; echo: large pericardial effusion

Tamponade

58-y/o male with Marfan syndrome presents with the abrupt onset of tearing chest pain radiating to the back; PE: ↓ BP, asymmetric pulses, declining mental status; CXR: widened mediastinum

Aortic dissection

70-y/o diabetic with hypercholesterolemia presents with angina, syncope, DOE; PE: diminished, slowly rising carotid pulses, crescendo-decrescendo systolic murmur at the second interspace at the right upper sternal border

Aortic stenosis

80-y/o diabetic with HTN and a h/o rheumatic heart disease presents with left-sided weakness; PE: pulses are irregularly irregular; ECG: absence of P waves and irregularly irregular QRS complexes

Atrial fibrillation (leading to embolic stroke)

70-y/o with a h/o CAD presents with worsening DOE, orthopnea, and paroxysmal nocturnal dyspnea; PE: JVD, S3 gallop, ⊕ hepatojugular reflex, bibasilar rales, and peripheral edema; CXR: cardiomegaly, bilateral pleural effusions

CHF

50-y/o chronic alcoholic presents with worsening DOE, orthopnea, and paroxysmal nocturnal dyspnea; PE: laterally displaced apical impulse; echocardiogram: four-chamber dilation, mitral and tricuspid regurgitation

Alcoholic dilated cardiomyopathy

35-y/o male with FH of sudden cardiac death presents with DOE and syncope; PE: double apical impulse, S4 gallop, holosystolic murmur at apex and axilla; echo: left ventricular hypertrophy and mitral regurgitation

Hypertrophic cardiomyopathy

40-y/o black male with h/o HTN presents with chest pain, dyspnea, and severe headache; PE: BP = 210/130 in all four extremities, flame-shaped retinal hemorrhages, papilledema; labs: negative vanillylmandelic acid (VMA) and urine catecholamines, and cardiac enzymes

Malignant HTN

15-y/o female presents 1 month after a sore throat with fever and joint pain. CBC shows leukocytosis. Labs: ASO+

Rheumatic fever

35-y/o female with a h/o rheumatic fever presents with worsening DOE and orthopnea; PE: loud S1, opening snap, and low-pitched diastolic murmur at the apex; CXR: left atrial enlargement

Mitral stenosis

65-y/o male presents with 1-h h/o substernal pressure and pain with radiation into the jaw and left arm, nausea, and diaphoresis; PE: S4 gallop; labs: ↑ troponin and CK-MB; ECG: ST elevation in leads aVL, V1-V4

Anterior MI

70-y/o female with DM and CAD presents with nausea and vomiting; PE: hypotension, clear lungs, JVD, right ventricular lift, and tricuspid valve regurgitation; ECG: ST elevation in the inferior leads

Right ventricular MI

40-y/o asymptomatic male; PE: displaced and diffuse apical impulse, diastolic murmur at left sternal border, brisk pulses with rapid collapse + "pistol shot" sound ascultated over large peripheral arteries

Aortic regurgitation

PULMONARY

Chronic Obstructive Pulmonary Disease

What are the classic PFT (pulmonary function test) values for obstructive lung disease?	FEV_1/FVC <80%
Name the type of obstructive pulmonary disease associated with the following features:	
Productive cough on most days during 3 or more consecutive months for 2 or more years that is worst in winter	Chronic bronchitis
Dyspnea and resultant hypertrophy of accessory muscles of inspiration	Emphysema
Cyanosis, rhonchi, wheezes, obesity, and signs of right-sided heart failure	Chronic bronchitis
Normal $Paco_2$, mildly ↓ Po_2	Emphysema
Hypertrophy/hyperplasia of mucus glands lining the airways	Chronic bronchitis
Destruction of alveolar walls leading to loss of elastic recoil and dilation of airspaces	Emphysema
Acute or subacute onset of dyspnea, expiratory wheezing, prolonged expiratory phase, accessory muscle use	Asthma
Pursed-lip breathing, prolonged expiratory phase	Emphysema
Commonly caused by cystic fibrosis (CF), severe/chronic pulmonary infection, or connective tissue disease	Bronchiectasis

Mucous plugging, airway smooth muscle hypertrophy, peripheral eosinophilia	Asthma
Barrel chest, ↓ breath sounds, hyperresonant to percussion	Emphysema
↑ $Paco_2$, ↓ Po_2, ↑ hematocrit (Hct) early in the course of disease	Chronic bronchitis
Lung hyperinflation on CXR	Emphysema, asthma
Airway irritability causing reversible bronchoconstriction; diagnose with methacholine challenge	Asthma
Permanent dilation of bronchioles	Bronchiectasis
Mildly ↓ Pao_2, respiratory alkalosis	Asthma
Halitosis, hemoptysis, and productive cough	Bronchiectasis
CXR may demonstrate subpleural blebs or parenchymal bullae.	Emphysema
Exacerbation may be triggered by cold air, exercise, inhaled dust, upper respiratory infection (URI), β-blockers, stress.	Asthma
CXR may show tram-track lung markings.	Bronchiectasis
What is the most beneficial lifestyle modification for a patient with chronic obstructive pulmonary disease (COPD)?	Smoking cessation
What prophylactic vaccines are recommended for patients with COPD?	Influenza and pneumococcal vaccines
What are the three classes of bronchodilators used for COPD and asthma?	1. $β_2$-Selective agonists, ie, albuterol 2. Anticholinergics, ie, ipratropium 3. Methylxanthine
What bronchodilator commonly used in COPD for relief of nocturnal symptoms can also cause nausea, vomiting, seizures, and arrhythmias?	Theophylline
What two classes of drugs are useful during acute COPD exacerbations?	1. Corticosteroids 2. Antibiotics

Which therapy can provide symptomatic relief and improve outcome in COPD patients with hypoxemia?	Supplemental oxygen therapy
What inherited disorder causes early progression of COPD?	α_1-Antitrypsin deficiency

Name the treatment of choice for the following clinical scenarios in an asthmatic:

First-line therapy for acute asthmatic attack	O_2, bronchodilators, steroids
Second-line therapy for acute asthmatic attack	$MgSO_4$ and intramuscular epinephrine
Initial therapy of mild asthma	Inhaled albuterol as needed
Mild asthma refractory to albuterol treatments	Inhaled glucocorticoids
Asthma attacks refractory to daily albuterol use	Systemic steroid therapy; usually with oral prednisone or IV methylprednisolone
Prophylaxis for asthma attacks (not including steroids)	Leukotriene inhibitors and cromolyn
Describe how glucocorticoids act on airways to control asthma:	↓ Inflammation and ↓ reactivity of airways to irritants (eg, cold, cigarette smoke, allergens, exercise)

Name the treatment for the following classes of asthmatic symptoms:

Mild intermittent	Daily treatment: none Quick relief: albuterol
Mild persistent	Daily treatment: low-dose steroids, isoniazid (INH) Quick relief: albuterol
Moderate persistent	Daily treatment: low-medium dose INH, long-acting β_2-selective agonist Quick relief: albuterol
Severe persistent	Daily treatment: high-dose steroid INH, long acting β_2-selective agonist, oral steroids Quick relief: albuterol

Restrictive Lung Disease

What are the classic PFTs for restrictive lung disease?

$FEV_1/FVC > 70\%$

Name the specific type of lung disease associated with the following descriptions:

65-y/o hay farmer with recent exposure to moldy hay presents with chronic dry cough, chest tightness; PE: bilateral diffuse rales; bronchoscopy: interstitial inflammation; bronchioalveolar lavage: lymphocyte and mast cell predominance

Hypersensitivity pneumonitis

35-y/o male presents with intermittent hemoptysis and hematuria; w/u: alveolar hemorrhage and acute GN

Goodpasture syndrome

40-y/o with progressive hypoxemia and cor pulmonale; lung biopsy: chronic inflammation of the alveolar wall in a pattern consistent with honeycomb lung; bronchioalveolar lavage: mild eosinophilia

Idiopathic pulmonary fibrosis

58-y/o former shipbuilder presents with the insidious onset of dyspnea; transbronchial biopsy demonstrates interstitial pulmonary fibrosis, ferruginous bodies; chest CT: demonstrates pleural effusion, and dense pleural fibrocalcific plaques

Asbestosis

55-y/o miner (nonsmoker) with dyspnea and dry cough; PFTs: obstructive and restrictive pattern; CXR: hilar lymphadenopathy with eggshell calcifications

Silicosis

60-y/o male with 100 pack-year h/o smoking presents with pleuritic chest pain, hemoptysis, and dyspnea; PE: dullness to percussion and absent breath sounds in the right lower lung field

Pleural effusion (2° to malignancy)

50-y/o former heavy smoker presents with multiple lung and rib lesions; excisional biopsy: lesions composed of cells (similar to the Langerhans cells of the skin) containing tennis racket—shaped Birbeck granules	Eosinophilic granuloma
30-y/o black female presents with DOE, fever, arthralgia; PE: iritis, erythema nodosum; labs: eosinophilia, ↑ serum ACE levels; PFT: restrictive pattern; CXR: bilateral hilar lymphadenopathy; lymph node biopsy: noncaseating granulomas	Sarcoidosis "GRAIN" Gammaglobulinemia Rhumetoid arthritis ACE increase Intersitial fibrosis Noncaseasting granulomas
How is the diagnosis of Lofgren syndrome (found in 25%-50%) made in sarcoidosis patients?	Hilar lymphadenopathy, polyarthralgias, and erthema nodosum
Name the four stages of sarcoidosis:	I. Hilar lymphadenopathy alone II. Lymphadenopathy + infiltrates III. Infiltrates alone IV. Fibrosis

Cystic Fibrosis

What are the common presenting symptoms of an infant with CF?	Meconium ileus, diarrhea, steatorrhea, malabsorption, failure to thrive, prolonged jaundice, recurrent URIs
What are the common presenting signs on examination of an infant with CF?	Cyanosis, clubbing, hyperresonant lung fields with occasional crackles, rectal prolapse, abdominal distention
What is the traditional diagnostic test for CF?	Sweat chloride test (⊕ if >60 mEq/L)
What is the definitive test for CF?	Genetic analysis
Which drugs are known to be beneficial in the management of CF?	Bronchodilators, antibiotics, and anti-inflammatory agents
What dietary supplements are necessary for patients with CF?	Pancreatic enzyme supplements and vitamins A, D, E, and K (the fat-soluble vitamins)
Which two methods are used to clear excess pulmonary secretions?	Physical therapy and DNAse therapy

Describe the effect of CF on each of the following organs:

Lungs

Recurrent pulmonary infections, bronchiesctasis. ↑ Residual volume (RV) and total lung capacity (TLC) in chronic disease; ↓ forced expiratory volume (FEV) in the first second (FEV_1)/FVC in acute exacerbation; pulmonary hemorrhage may occur

Pancreas

Variable defects in pancreatic exocrine function; may cause pancreatic insufficiency, fatty stool, weight loss

Intestines

Mucus plugs → small bowel obstruction; meconium ileus in some infants

Salivary glands

Ductal dilation; squamous metaplasia of ductal epithelium and glandular atrophy

Liver

Plugging of bile canaliculi → cirrhosis

Epididymis and ductus deferens

Obstruction → azospermia and infertility

What is the classic finding on pulmonary examination in a patient with idiopathic pulmonary fibrosis?

Fine expiratory crackles (*velcro crackles*)

How does interstitial lung disease affect alveolar gas diffusion and lung volumes?

Interstitial fibrosis decreases gas diffusion and lung volumes.

Which group of interstitial lung diseases can present with a combination of obstructive and restrictive pattern on PFTs?

Pneumoconioses

Which group of interstitial lung diseases is caused by a deposition of immune complexes in the alveoli and granuloma formation?

Hypersensitivity pneumonitis

Name several commonly used drugs that are known to cause interstitial lung disease:

Bleomycin, vincristine, alkylating agents, and amiodarone

What are typical findings on CXR in a patient with interstitial lung disease?

Reticular or reticulonodular infiltrates or honeycomb lung

Name the interstitial lung disease(s) with the following findings on CXR:

Bilateral linear opacities and broad pleural plaques	Asbestosis
Nodular opacities in the upper lung zones	Coal worker's pneumoconiosis, silicosis
Diffuse infiltrates in the upper lung zones	Berylliosis, hypersensitivity pneumonitis

Patients with silicosis are at increased risk for which infectious disease?

Tuberculosis

What is the definitive diagnostic test for interstitial lung diseases?

Biopsy

What are the two general principles of treatment for hypersensitivity pneumonitis and the pneumoconioses?

1. Corticosteroids
2. Prevention of exposure to offending agents

What is the mainstay of treatment for patients with sarcoidosis?

Corticosteroids

Pleural Effusion

Name the type of pleural effusion (transudate, exudate, or both) associated with the following features:

Common presentation includes dyspnea, pleuritic chest pain, hemoptysis, cough.	Both
Pathophysiologic mechanism is based on a breakdown of the pleural membrane and capillaries.	Exudate
Due to excess production or inadequate reabsorption of pleural fluid	Both
Pathophysiologic mechanism is based on changes in Starling's forces.	Transudate
Decreased breath sounds, ↓ tactile fremitus, and dullness to percussion in the region of the effusion	Both
Effusion containing bacteria	Exudate
Commonly caused by cirrhosis, nephrotic syndrome, protein losing enteropathy, or heart failure	Transudate

Commonly caused by malignancy, tuberculosis, infection, SLE, rheumatoid arthritis (RA)	Exudate
May be caused by a PE	Both
pH <7.2, glucose <50	Exudate
(Pleural lactate dehydrogenase [LDH])/(serum LDH) >0.6	Exudate
(Pleural protein)/(serum protein) <0.5	Transudate
Specific gravity of effusion >1.015	Exudate
Name three conditions which may lead to a pleural effusion containing amylase:	1. Pancreatitis 2. Esophageal rupture (traumatic or postoperative) 3. Malignancy
What term is used to describe an exudative pulmonary effusion which contains gross pus, has readily visible bacteria, has a glucose <50, or a pH <7?	Empyema (complicated parapneumonic effusion)
What type of analysis should be performed on a patient in which malignancy is thought to be the cause of a pleural effusion?	Cytology
What class of drugs is often used to treat a transudative effusion?	Diuretics
What procedure is performed to prevent reaccumulation of a malignant pleural effusion?	Pleurodesis
In addition to antibiotic coverage for pneumonia, what is the appropriate management for an empyema?	Chest tube drainage
What diagnosis is suggested by pleural fluid containing RBC >100,000 in the absence of trauma or pulmonary infarction?	Pleural malignancy

Pulmonary Embolism

What is the incidence of PE in autopsies?	Greater than 50%
What is the incidence of PE in hospitalized patients?	20%-25%

What is the etiology of 95% of pulmonary emboli?

Dislodged lower extremity deep venous thromboses (DVT)

What is the most common clinical presentation of PE?

Sinus tachycardia

What are the other common presenting symptoms of PE?

Fever, pleuritic chest pain, cough, dyspnea/tachypnea, swollen and painful leg, and anxiety

What factors favor the development of a DVT?

Virchow's triad
1. Stasis
2. Hypercoagulability
3. Endothelial dysfunction

What are the two most common CXR findings in a patient with PE?

1. Normal CXR
2. Cardiomegaly

What are the *classic* CXR findings in a patient with a PE?

Pleural effusion, Hampton's hump (a distal wedge-shaped infarct), and Westermark's sign (hyperlucency in the region of lung supplied by the infarcted artery)

What is the most common ECG finding in a patient with PE?

Sinus tachycardia

What is the classic ECG finding in a patient with PE?

S1Q3T3 (S wave in lead I, Q wave and *inverted* T in lead III)

What are modified Well's criteria for DVT/PE risk stratification?

3 points each: no Dx more likely, physical signs of DVT (asymmetric LE edema)

1.5 points each: tachycardia, hospitalized in past month/surgery, past hx of DVT

1 point each: hemoptysis, malignancy

0-1 = low risk (rule out w/ neg D-dimer)

2-6 = intermediate risk

>7 = high risk (treat w/ positive LE Doppler US)

What two diagnostic tests are commonly used to diagnose PE?

1. Chest CT with contrast
2. Ventilation/perfusion scan (when contrast is contraindicated)

What is the gold standard test for diagnosis of PE?

Pulmonary angiogram

What serologic test can assist in ruling out PE when negative in low-risk patients?

D-dimer

What thrombolytic drug may be used in massive PE causing hemodynamic instability?	Tissue plasminogen activator (t-PA)
What therapy is indicated for high-risk patients during the w/u of PE and for patients diagnosed with PE?	IV heparin
What are the contraindications for anticoagulation with heparin?	1. h/o heparin-induced thrombocytopenia (HITS) 2. Intracranial hemorrhage or neoplasm 3. Recent major surgery 4. Bleeding diathesis
Why should heparin be continued for several days after warfarin therapy is begun?	1. Warfarin takes several days to become therapeutic. 2. Initially warfarin induces a hypercoagulable state (by inactivating proteins C and S), which may cause skin necrosis.
What methods are used for long-term prophylaxis for patients at risk of developing DVT?	Warfarin or IVC filter
What is an alternative to warfarin for outpatient DVT prophylaxis?	Low-molecular-weight heparin
What type of tumors commonly cause a DVT by inducing a hypercoagulable state?	Adenocarcinomas
What commonly used medication increases the risk of DVT?	Oral contraceptives
What is the most common genetic disease that predisposes to the development of DVT?	Factor V Leiden

Pulmonary Edema

What syndrome is suggested by the presence of acute, refractory hypoxemia, decreased lung compliance, and pulmonary edema in a patient with normal pulmonary capillary wedge pressure?	Acute respiratory distress syndrome (ARDS)

What syndrome is suggested by the presence of pulmonary edema in a patient with an elevated pulmonary capillary wedge pressure?	Cardiogenic pulmonary edema
What are the diagnostic criteria for ARDS?	1. Acute onset of respiratory distress 2. $PaO_2/FIO_2 \leq 200$ 3. Bilateral pulmonary infiltrates on CXR 4. Normal capillary wedge pressure
What is the most common risk factor for ARDS?	Sepsis
Name five additional common risk factors for ARDS:	Lung injury due to aspiration of gastric contents, trauma, pancreatitis, drug overdose, shock
What type of respiratory therapy is indicated in ARDS?	Mechanical ventilation

Pneumothorax

What are the two most common presenting symptoms in spontaneous pneumothorax (PTX)?	Unilateral chest pain and dyspnea
What are the common presenting signs in a patient with spontaneous PTX?	Tachypnea, unilateral diminished/absent breath sounds, and hyperresonance to percussion
What is the most common cause of primary spontaneous PTX?	Rupture of subpleural apical bullae
What are the most common causes of 2° spontaneous PTX?	COPD (most common), CF, pulmonary infections (especially PCP pneumonia and TB), trauma, and iatrogenic
What widely used ICU procedure carries the risk of PTX?	Placement of subclavian or internal jugular central venous catheters
What are the common presenting signs in a patient with tension PTX?	Dyspnea, tachypnea, jugular venous distention, hemodynamic instability, and lateral displacement of trachea
What is the appearance of a PTX on CXR?	Pleural stripe with absent lung markings

What are the classic findings on CXR in tension PTX?	Hyperlucent lung field (ipsilateral), depressed diaphragm (ipsilateral), tracheal and mediastinal deviation (away from PTX), and compression of the contralateral lung
What is the treatment of a spontaneous PTX?	**Asymptomatic** → observation and O_2 therapy; **symptomatic** → may require chest tube drainage
What is the management of a tension PTX?	Emergent needle thoracostomy at the second interspace at the midclavicular line
Which patients with PTX get tube thoracostomy?	Symptomatic patients or PTX 2/2 underlying lung disease
Which patients with PTX are treated with needle aspiration?	Those with minimal dyspnea, < age 50, small (<2 cm) PTX

Pneumonia

What is the common presentation of typical (bacterial) pneumonia?	Fever >39°C (102.2°F), chills, cough productive of blood tinged, purulent sputum, and pleuritic pain (acute onset)
What is the common presentation of atypical "walking" pneumonia?	Fever <39°C (102.2°F), nonproductive cough, headache, and GI upset (insidious onset)
What are the common physical findings in pneumonia?	Bronchial breath sounds, crackles, wheezes, egophany, dullness to percussion, and tactile fremitus
What is the classic CXR finding in typical pneumonia?	Lobar consolidation
What is the classic CXR finding in atypical pneumonia?	Patchy alveolar infiltrates
Name the most common organism(s) causing the following pulmonary infection:	
Lobar pneumonia	*Streptococcus pneumoniae*
Bronchopneumonia	*S. aureus* and *Haemophilus influenza*
Interstitial pneumonia	*Mycoplasma pneumoniae* (most common), *Legionella pneumophila*, and *Chlamydia pneumonia*

Fungal pneumonia in AIDS patient with CD4$^+$ count <200	*Pneumocystis jiroveci*
Typical pneumonia in neonate	*Streptococcus agalactiae*
Alcoholic with typical pneumonia after aspiration	*Klebsiella pneumoniae*
Atypical pneumonia in younger patient with positive cold agglutinin test	*M. pneumoniae*
Neonate with atypical pneumonia and trachoma	*Chlamydia trachomatis*
Dairy worker with atypical pneumonia	*Coxiella burnetti*
Rabbit hunter with atypical pneumonia	*Francisella tularensis*
Pet bird owner with pneumonia, splenomegaly, bradycardia	*Chlamydia psittaci*
Hospitalized patient with lobar pneumonia	*S. pneumoniae* > *S. aureus*
IV drug user with pneumonia	*S. pneumoniae, K. pneumoniae,* and *S. aureus*
Patient recovering from viral URI	*S. aureus* and *H. influenza*
Chicken farmer from the Ohio river valley with atypical pneumonia	*Histoplasma capsulatum*
Patient from southwestern United States with atypical pneumonia	*Coccidioides immitis*
Most common cause of community-acquired pneumonia	*S. pneumoniae*
Best treated with naficillin, oxacillin, methicillin, or vancomycin (for penicillin-resistant strains)	*S. aureus*
Causes severe pneumonia in CF patients and readily develops multidrug resistance	*Pseudomonas* spp.
Cough productive of dark red, mucoid, currant jelly sputum production in an alcoholic or diabetic	*K. pneumoniae*
Rust-colored sputum	*S. pneumoniae*

Lobar pneumonia in a smoker with COPD; sputum with gram-negative rods and many leukocytes; best treated with macrolides	*H. influenzae*
Recommended treatment includes third-generation cephalosporin or fluoroquinolone	Gram-negative rods: *Pseudomonas* spp., *K. pneumoniae, and H. influenzae*
Pneumonia following influenza infection	*S. aureus*
Associated with inhalation of contaminated water droplets from air conditioners	*L. pneumophila*
Lung abscess with air/fluid level on CXR	*S. aureus*
Pneumonia accompanied by hyponatremia, mental status changes, diarrhea, and LDH >700	*L. pneumophila*
Gram-positive, weakly acid-fast organism causing pneumonia in patients with AIDS; associated with peripheral eosinophilia	*Nocardia asteroides*
Fungus ball on CXR	*Aspergillus*
Name the most common causative pathogen(s) of pneumonia for each of the following age group:	
Neonates	Group B streptococci, *Escherichia coli,* and *C. pneumoniae*
Children (6 weeks to 18 years)	Respiratory syncytial virus (RSV) and other viruses, *M. pneumoniae, C. pneumoniae,* and *S. pneumoniae*
Adults (18-40 years old)	*M. pneumoniae, C. pneumoniae,* and *S. pneumoniae*
Adults (45-65 years old)	*S. pneumoniae, H. influenzae,* anaerobes, viruses, and *M. pneumoniae*
Adults (>65 years old)	*S. pneumoniae,* viruses, anaerobes, *H. influenzae,* and gram-negative rods

List the appropriate empiric therapy
and most common organisms causing
pneumonia in each of the following
scenarios:

Community-acquired pneumonia in
a healthy patient <60 y/o

Empiric therapy: macrolide
(Azithromycin), fluoroquinolone
(Levofloxacin), or tetracycline
(Doxycycline)

Organisms: *S. pneumoniae, M. pneumoniae,
C. pneumoniae, H. influenzae,* and
respiratory viruses

Community-acquired pneumonia
in a healthy patient >60 y/o or
with comorbidities (CHF, COPD,
DM, alcoholic, renal or
liver failure)

Empiric therapy: Second-generation
cephalosporin (eg, cefuroxime) and
amoxicillin; add erythromycin if
atypical pathogens are suspected

Organisms: *S. pneumoniae, H. influenzae,*
aerobic gram-negative bacilli, *S. aureus,*
and respiratory viruses

Community-acquired pneumonia in
a patient requiring hospitalization

Empiric therapy: antipneumococcal
fluoroquinolone IV

Organisms: *S. pneumoniae* (including
resistant strains), *H. influenzae, M.
pneumoniae, C. pneumoniae,*
polymicrobial

Community-acquired pneumonia in
a patient requiring ICU admission

Empiric therapy: antipseudomonal
β-lactam (eg, cefepime) plus an
antipseudomonal quinolone
(eg, ciprofloxacin) all IV

Organisms: *S. pneumoniae* (including
resistant strains), *Legionella* spp.,
H. influenzae, enteric gram-negative
bacilli, *S. aureus,* and *P. aeruginosa*

Hospital-acquired pneumonia

Vancomycin, Cefepime, and
ciprofloxacin

Which patients are at risk for
ventilator-associated pneumonia
(VAP)?

Patients with chest trauma, GCS < 9,
and mechanical ventilation

What can be done to help prevent VAP?

Raise head of bed >45°, maintain gastric
acid, maximize nutrition, prevent
colonization by healthcare workers, and
use respiratory equipment in a sterile
fashion

Which patients should receive the
pneumococcal vaccine?

Patients >65 y/o and
immunocompromised patients
(including postsplenectomy and sickle
cell patients)

Name four common complications of lobar pneumonia:	1. Abscess formation (especially *S. aureus* and anaerobes) 2. Empyema or spread of infection to the pleural cavity 3. Organization of exudate to form scar tissue 4. Sepsis
What type of infection is characterized by localized suppurative necrosis of lung tissue?	Lung abscess
Name several bacterial pathogens capable of causing lung abscess:	*Staphylococci, streptococci,* gram-negative bacilli, anaerobes, and oral flora
Name the two bacterial pathogens commonly associated with lobar pneumonia complicated by empyema:	*S. pneumoniae > S. aureus*

Pulmonary Neoplasms

What is the most common cause of cancer deaths in the United States for both males and females?	Lung cancer
What is the most common type of malignant lung tumor?	Metastasic lesions
What are the most common primary lung tumors?	Adenocarcinoma and squamous cell carcinoma (equal incidence)
What are the common presenting symptoms of lung cancer?	Cough, hemoptysis, dyspnea, chest pain, constitutional symptoms
Name the type(s) of primary lung cancer associated with the following features:	
Central location	"Sentral" is Squamous cell and Small (oat) cell carcinomas
Peripheral location	Adenocarcinoma, large cell, and bronchioalveolar carcinoma
Commonly found within large bronchi	Squamous cell and small (oat) cell carcinomas
Clear link to smoking	Squamous cell
No clear link to smoking	Bronchoalveolar adenocarcinoma
Most malignant tumor (often metastatic at diagnosis)	Small (oat) cell carcinoma

Often secretes parathyroid hormone (PTH)-related peptide	Squamous cell carcinoma
Associated with production of ADH and ACTH	Small (oat) cell carcinoma
Carcinoembryonic antigen (CEA) ⊕	Adenocarcinoma
Secretion of 5-HT results in tachycardia, diarrhea, skin flushing, wheezing.	Carcinoid
Tumor cells lining alveolar walls	Bronchioloalveolar adenocarcinoma
Giant pleomorphic cells, many cerebral metastasis, poor prognosis	Large cell
Associated with dermatomyositis, acanthosis nigricans	All types
Associated with peripheral neuropathy and Lambert-Eaton myasthenic syndrome	Small (oat) cell carcinoma
Associated with thrombophlebitis and marantic endocarditis	Adenocarcinoma

In each of the following clinical scenarios, name the structure being compressed or irritated by a lung tumor:

Cough	Phrenic nerve
Hoarseness	Recurrent laryngeal nerve
Facial and upper extremity swelling	Superior vena cava (SVC) syndrome
Ptosis, miosis, hemianhydrosis	Sympathetic cervical ganglion (Horner syndrome)

What percentage of solitary pulmonary nodules is malignant?	40%
What is the differential diagnosis for a solitary pulmonary nodule?	Infectious granuloma, carcinoma, benign neoplasm, bronchial adenoma, and pneumonia
Are routine CXRs a good way to screen for lung cancer/carcinoma (CA)?	No
What is an effective way to lower the risk of lung CA?	Smoking cessation
What is the treatment for small cell carcinoma?	Radiation and chemotherapy
What is the treatment for nonsmall cell carcinoma that is local?	Tumor resection and radiation therapy

What is the treatment for nonsmall cell carcinoma that has metastasized?	Radiation and chemotherapy
What rare pleural tumor is found in patients with a h/o occupational exposure to asbestos?	Malignant mesothelioma

Decide whether the following features of a solitary pulmonary nodule favor a *benign* or *malignant* etiology:

Age >40 years	Malignant
Size >2 cm	Malignant
Well-circumscribed mass	Benign
Absence of calcification or irregular calcification	Malignant
Growth in lesion from previous CXRs	Malignant
Central, uniform, or laminated calcification	Benign

Make the Diagnosis

7-y/o with h/o environmental allergies presents in acute respiratory distress; PE: ↑ tachypnea expiratory wheezes, intercostal retractions, accessory muscle use; CXR: hyperinflation; complete blood count (CBC) shows eosinophilia

Bronchial asthma

60-y/o with a 50 pack-year h/o smoking presents with fever and cough productive of thick sputum for the past 4 months; PE: cyanosis, crackles, wheezes; w/u: Hct = 48, WBC = 12,000; CXR: no infiltrates

Chronic bronchitis

60-y/o with a 50 pack-year h/o smoking presents with DOE and dry cough but no chest pain; PE: ↓ breath sounds, hyperresonant chest, ↑ heart rate (HR), distant S1 and S2; CXR: flattened diaphragm.

Emphysema

60-y/o with 50 pack-year h/o smoking presents with fatigue, dyspnea, hoarseness, anorexia; PE: miosis, ptosis, anhydrosis, and dullness to percussion at right apex; chest CT: large hilar mass extending into the right superior pulmonary sulcus

Pancoast tumor, (most likely bronchogenic squamous cell carcinoma, causing Horner syndrome)

60-y/o patient in days 4 status post (s/p) total knee replacement has the sudden onset of tachycardia, tachypnea, sharp chest pain, hypotension; arterial blood gas (ABG): respiratory alkalosis; ECG: sinus tachycardia; venous duplex US: clot in right femoral vein

Pulmonary embolus

40-y/o white male presents with chronic rhinosinusitis, ear pain, cough, dyspnea; PE: ulcerations of nasal mucosa, perforation of nasal septum; w/u: ↑ (c-ANCA), red cell casts in urine; biopsy of nasal lesions: necrotizing vasculitis and granulomas

Wegener's granulomatosis

50-y/o obese male with resistant hypertension complaining of morning headache, awakening without feeling refreshed, and daytime sleepiness

Obstructive sleep apnea

55-y/o female presents with dyspnea and nonproductive cough; PE: "velcro-like" basilar end-inspiratory crackles and clubbing; CXR: basilar infiltrates; PFTs: FEV_1/ FVC >70%, ↓ DLCO

Idiopathic pulmonary fibrosis

40-y/o African American woman presents with dyspnea and polyarthritis; PE: acute, nodular erythematous eruption on extensor surface of lower extremities; CXR: hilar lymphadenopathy; biopsy would show noncaseating granuloma with no infection

Sarcoidosis

INFECTIOUS DISEASES

Fever

Name the six "do-not-miss" diagnoses of infections that present with fever and rash:	1. Meningococcemia 2. Bacterial sepsis (eg, *Staphylococcus*) 3. Endocarditis 4. Gonococcemia 5. Rocky Mountain spotted fever (RMSF) 6. Typhoid fever
What criteria are used to define fever of unknown origin (FUO)?	Temperature >38.3°C (101°F) for >3 weeks with failure to diagnose (despite 1 week of inpatient investigation or several outpatient visits)

Name three common causes of FUO
for each of the following categories:

    Infectious (30%-40% of cases)   Endocarditis, TB, and occult abscess (usually abdominal)

    Neoplastic (20%-30% of cases)   Leukemia, lymphoma, and renal cell CA

    Autoimmune (15%-20% of cases)   Giant cell arteritis, polymyalgia rheumatica, and juvenile RA

Ear, Nose, and Throat Infections

Name four risk factors for sinusitis?
1. Smoking
2. Viral infection
3. Allergies
4. Barotrauma

What are the most common bacterial pathogens causing acute sinusitis?

S. pneumoniae, H. influenzae, and *Moraxella catarrhalis*

What sinuses are most commonly involved in acute sinusitis?

Maxillary sinuses (drain superiorly against gravity)

Name three key clinical findings of acute sinusitis:
1. Purulent rhinorrhea
2. Facial pain
3. Maxillary tooth pain

What is the treatment of acute sinusitis lasting >2 weeks?

Bactrim, amoxicillin, doxycycline (10 days PO), and decongestants

What condition results from obstruction of sinus drainage and ongoing anaerobic infection?

Chronic sinusitis

What is the treatment of chronic sinusitis?

6-12 weeks PO antibiotics; surgical correction of obstruction for refractory cases

Diabetics are at increased risk for developing what type of severe sinusitis?

Mucormycosis

Name four potential complications of sinusitis:
1. Meningitis
2. Frontal bone osteomyelitis
3. Abscess formation
4. Cavernous sinus thrombosis

Where do the majority of bleeds from epistaxis occur?

Kiesselbach plexus (anterior nasal septum)

What is the most common cause of epistaxis in kids?

Exploration with digits

What are the two most common pathogens causing otitis externa (*swimmer's ear*)?	1. *Pseudomonas* 2. Enterobacteriaceae
What PE finding is virtually pathognomonic for otitis externa?	Pulling on pinna or pushing tragus causes pain.
What is the treatment of choice for otitis externa?	Antibiotic eardrops (dicloxacillin for acute disease)
What group of patients is at ↑ risk for complications from otitis externa?	Diabetics— ↑ risk of malignant otitis externa and osteomyelitis of temporal bone/skull base

Name the responsible organism and treatment for each of the following types of pharyngitis:

Fever, sore throat, and red eye	Adenovirus
Oral thrush; seen in AIDS and small kids	Fungus (*Candida*)
Pathognomonic gray membranes on tonsils	Diphtheria (membranous pharyngitis)
High fever, sore throat with exudative tonsillitis, and cervical lymphadenopathy; cough usually absent	Group A *Streptococcus*
Tonsillitis, splenomegaly, palatal petechiae, and posterior auricular lymphadenopathy	Epstein-Barr virus (EBV) (mononucleosis)

Tuberculosis

Decide whether each statement is more closely associated with 1° or 2° tuberculosis (TB):

Classically affects lower lobes	Primary TB
Associated with reactivation	2° TB
Fibrocaseous cavitary lung lesion	2° TB
Ghon complex on CXR	Primary TB
Affects apical lungs (↑ affinity for ↑ O_2 environment)	2° TB
Presents with cough/hemoptysis, fever, night sweats, weight loss	2° TB

What is the primary mode of transmission of *Mycobacterium tuberculosis*?

Respiratory droplets

What term is used to describe the lymphatic and hematogenous spread of TB, causing numerous small foci of infection in extrapulmonary sites?

Miliary TB

Name the five most common sites of extrapulmonary TB:

1. Central nervous system (CNS) (tuberculous meningitis)
2. Vertebral bodies (Pott disease)
3. Psoas major muscle → abscess
4. Liver
5. Cervical lymph nodes → scrofuloderma (massive lymphadenopathy)

How is active TB infection diagnosed?

Clinical and radiologic signs of 2° TB and acid-fast bacilli in sputum

What is an effective screening tool for latent TB?

Purified protein derivative (PPD) test

What constitutes a positive PPD test?

>5-mm induration for HIV⊕ or immunocompromised individuals

>10-mm induration for high-risk individuals

>15-mm induration for anyone else

What condition often causes a false negative PPD?

Immunosuppression → check anergy panel

What is the management of PPD ⊕ latent TB?

Treatment with isoniazid (INH) for 9 months

What is the management for active TB?

Respiratory isolation, initial four-drug therapy: "RIPE": **R**ifampin, **I**NH, **P**yrizinamide, **E**thambutol → narrowed when sensitivities determined (treat for >6 months)

Note: give vitamin B_6 with INH.

What is the major toxicity of many TB drugs?

Hepatotoxicity; check LFTs if symptomatic or h/o liver disease

Human Immunodeficiency Virus

What test is used to rule out the diagnosis of human immunodeficiency virus **(HIV) because of its high sensitivity?**

Enzyme-linked immunosorbent assay (ELISA) (to detect antibodies [Ab] to viral proteins)

What test is used to confirm a positive HIV test because of its high specificity?

Western blot assay (high false negative within 2 months of infection)

What are the common presenting signs of the viral prodrome of HIV, ie, acute retroviral syndrome?

Fever (97%), fatigue (90%), lymphadenopathy (50%-77%), pharyngitis (73%), transient rash (40%-70%), or headache (30%-60%)

How is AIDS defined?

$CD4^+$ <200 cells/mL or serologic evidence of AIDS-defining illness

What mutation may confer resistance to infection with HIV?

Homozygous deletion of CCR5 (or other viral receptors)

Name the AIDS opportunistic infection or disease associated with the following:

Fungal

Candida (thrush), *Cryptococcus* (meningitis), *P. jeroveci* pneumonia, histoplasmosis, and coccidioidosis

Bacterial

M. tuberculosis (TB), *Staphylococcus*, encapsulated organisms, and *M. avium-intracellulare* (MAC complex)

Viral

Herpes simplex virus (HSV), varicella-zoster virus (VZV) (shingles), cytomegalovirus (CMV) (retinitis), JC virus (PML), Epstein-Barr virus (EBV) (B-cell lymphoma), and human herpesvirus (HHV)-8 (Kaposi sarcoma)

Protozoal

Toxoplasma (encephalopathy), and *Cryptosporidium* (severe watery diarrhea)

State the typical $CD4^+$ count associated with each of the following HIV complications:

TB becomes more common

<400 cells/mL

Serious opportunists are first seen

<200 cells/mL

Toxoplasmosis, cryptococcosis

<100 cells/mL

MAC, CMV, and cryptosporidiosis

<50 cells/mL

What constitutes highly active antiretroviral therapy (HAART)?

Two nucleoside RT inhibitors combined with protease inhibitor or nonnucleoside RT inhibitor

Note: no patient should ever be on monotherapy due to the risk of resistance.

What test is used to monitor the effectiveness of antiretroviral therapy?	HIV polymerase chain reaction (PCR) (measures viral load)
Name the medical management for the following HIV⊕ patients:	
CD4$^+$ <500 or detectable viral load	Initiate HAART
CD4$^+$ <200	Bactrim prophylaxis for PCP
CD4$^+$ <75	Azithromycin prophylaxis for MAC
CD4$^+$ <50	Fluconazole prophylaxis for fungi
Pregnant HIV⊕ patient	Zidovudine (azidothymidine [AZT])—↓ vertical transmission
State the treatment of choice for immunocompromised patients with influenza:	Prevention: trivalent inactivated influenza vaccine Post-exposure prophylaxis: zanamivir or oseltamivir
Why is oseltamivir preferred in asthmatics in the treatment of influenza?	Zanamivir is associated with bronchospasm in 5%-10% of patients with asthma.

Urinary Tract Infections

Name six risk factors for urinary tract infections (UTIs):	1. Foley catheter 2. Diabetes mellitus 3. Anatomic anomaly 4. Pregnancy 5. ↑ Sexual activity 6. H/o UTI or pyelonephritis
Name three common presenting symptoms in UTI:	1. Frequency 2. Dysuria 3. Urgency
What two clinical findings suggest pyelonephritis?	1. Fever 2. Back/flank pain
What is the most common presenting symptom in a child with a UTI?	Bedwetting
Why are women at ten times the risk of men for developing a UTI?	The urethra is shorter in women and more likely to be colonized with fecal flora.

Name the specific urinary finding
associated with each of the
following:

Microscopic analysis in UTI
>5 WBC/high-power field

Urine dipstick in UTI
↑ Leukocyte esterace, ↑ nitrites (specific
for gram negatives)

Clean-catch urine culture in a UTI
>100,000 CFU/mL of bacteria

Characteristic urinalysis (UA)
finding in *Proteus* infection
↑ Urine pH

Characteristic UA finding
in cystitis
Hematuria

Characteristic UA finding in acute
pyelonephritis
WBC casts

List the most common UTI organisms:
"SEEKS PP"

Serratia marcescens

E. coli

Enterobacter cloacae

K. pneumoniae

Staphylococcus saprophyticus

Proteus mirabilis

P. aeruginosa

Which UTI-causing bug is frequently
nosocomial, drug-resistant, and may
produce a red pigment?
S. marcescens

What is the first-line antibiotic for
lower UTIs?
Bactrim (trimethoprim [TMP]-
sulfamethoxazole [SMX]) for 3 days;
amoxicillin for *Enterococcus*

What is the treatment for pylonephritis?
Levofloxacin PO 7 days (IV if pt has
nausea/vomiting).

Sexually Transmitted Diseases

Name the sexually transmitted disease
(STD) associated with the following
descriptions and provide the treatment
of choice:

Clue cells in Pap smear; positive
"whiff test"
Bacterial vaginosis (eg, *Gardnerella
vaginitis*)

Tx: Flagyl (metronidazole)

Soft, painful sexually transmitted ulcer associated with inguinal lymphadenopathy	Chancroid (caused by *Haemophilus ducreyi)* **Tx:** ceftriaxone, ciprofloxacin, or erythromycin
Raised, red papules; biopsy shows Donovan bodies	Granuloma inguinale (caused by *Calymmatobacterium granulomatis)* **Tx:** doxycycline 100 mg bid × 3 weeks
Firm, painless chancre caused by a spirochete	Syphilis (caused by *Treponema pallidum*) Tx: Penicillin G
Most common STD; frequent cause of pelvic inflammatory disease (PID) in women and urethritis in men; associated with Reiter syndrome	Chlamydial cervicitis (types D-K) **Tx:** azithromycin; erythromycin in pregnancy; treat presumptive gonorrhea coinfection
Small papule/ulcer that leads to enlargement of lymph nodes; caused by *C. trachomatis* serotypes L1, L2, or L3	Lymphogranuloma venereum **Tx:** same as for Chlamydial cervicitis
STD that can result in extragenital infections (eg, pharyngitis, proctitis, arthritis, and neonatal conjunctivitis)	Gonorrhea (caused by *Neisseria gonorrhoeae*) **Tx:** ceftriaxone; treat presumptive chlamydia coinfection
STD resulting in benign venereal warts caused by human papillomavirus (HPV) types 6 and 11	Condyloma acuminatum **Tx:** cryotherapy or topical podophyllin
Painful vesicles/ulcers; cytology shows multinuclear giant cells; diagnose with Tzanck prep	Herpes genitalis (most often HSV type 2) **Tx:** acyclovir (for 1° infection or suppression)
STD caused by flagellated, motile protozoan; #2 cause of vaginitis	Trichomoniasis **Tx:** flagyl (metronidazole)

Name the stage of syphilis associated with each of the following descriptions:

Rash on palms and soles with lymphadenopathy	2° syphilis
Firm, painless chancre	1° syphilis
After 1 year of infection; can progress to 3° syphilis	Late latent
First year of infection; no symptoms, but positive serology	Early latent
Tabes dorsalis, aortitis, Argyll-Robertson pupil, gummas	3° syphilis

Name three tests that can be used to diagnose syphilis:	1. Dark-field microscopy (visible spirochetes) 2. VDRL/RPR (fast, cheap, nonspecific) 3. Fluorescent treponemal antibody—absorbed (FTA-ABS) (sensitive, specific, positive for life)
What is the treatment for syphilis?	Penicillin (IV for neurosyphilis); $\uparrow$ dose by 3× if undiagnosed for >1 year
What complication of syphilis treatment results in fever and flu-like symptoms caused by the massive destruction of spirochetes?	Jarisch-Herxheimer reaction

Osteomyelitis

What are the two main routes of infection for osteomyelitis?	1. Direct spread (80%) 2. Hematogenous seeding (20%)
Where does hematogenous osteomyelitis typically occur?	Metaphyses of long bones in children ($\uparrow$ vascularity of growth plates); vertebral bodies of IV drug abusers

Name the organism typically responsible for osteomyelitis in each of the following situations:

Newborn	*Streptococci* spp. or *E. coli*
Child	*Staphylococcus aureus*
Otherwise healthy adult	*S. aureus*
Foot puncture wound	*Pseudomonas* spp.
Intravenous drug user	*Pseudomonas* spp. or *S. aureus*
Sickle cell disease	*Salmonella* spp.
Hip replacement (or other prosthesis)	*Staphylococcus epidermidis*
Chronic osteomyelitis	*S. aureus, Pseudomonas* spp., *Enterobacteriaceae*
Asplenic patient	*Salmonella* spp.

What is the classic radiographic finding in osteomyelitis?	Periosteal elevation

What is the gold standard for evaluation of osteomyelitis?	MRI (can confirm with bone aspiration and culture)
What is the treatment regimen for pyogenic osteomyelitis?	6-8 weeks of antibiotics; fluoroquinolones empirically → narrow as cultures come back; surgical debridement if necessary
Name four complications of osteomyelitis:	1. Chronic osteomyelitis 2. Septic arthritis 3. Systemic sepsis 4. Draining sinus tract → squamous cell carcinoma

Vector-borne Illness

What is the most common vector-borne disease in the United States?	Lyme disease
Name the organism and the vector involved in Lyme disease:	*Borrelia burgdorferi* is carried by *Ixodes* ticks.
What is the treatment for Lyme disease?	Ceftriaxone, high-dose penicillin, or doxycycline
Name the stage of Lyme disease associated with each of the following classic PE findings:	
Migratory polyarthropathy/arthralgias, meningitis, myocarditis (with conduction defects), neurologic problems	2° Lyme disease
Erythema chronicum migrans	Primary Lyme disease
Encephalitis and arthritis	Tertiary (3°) Lyme disease
Which tick-borne disease can lead to small vessel vasculitis?	RMSF
Name the organism and the vector involved in RMSF:	*Rickettsia rickettsii* is carried by Dermacentor tick.
Name four common PE findings in RMSF:	1. Fever 2. Headache 3. Myalgias 4. Classic maculopapular rash (begins on palms/soles → spreads centrally)

What is the differential diagnosis for a rash affecting the palms and soles?	RMSF, 2° syphilis, hand-foot-mouth disease (coxsackie A), and Kawasaki syndrome
What is the treatment for RMSF?	Doxycycline; chloramphenicol in pregnant women and kids

Sepsis

Define sepsis?	An infection that causes systemic inflammatory response syndrome (SIRS)
Define SIRS?	Two or more of the following: 1. T > 38.0°C (100.4°F) or < 36.0°C (96.8°F) 2. HR >90 3. RR >20 or P_{CO_2} <32 mm Hg 4. WBC >12,000 or < 4000 or >10% band forms
What type of bacteria cause shock through endotoxin-mediated vasodilation?	Gram-negative bacteria

Name the organism(s) that most commonly cause sepsis in the following groups:

IV drug abusers	*S. aureus*
Asplenic/sickle cell patients	Encapsulated bacteria (*H. influenzae, Meningococcus, Pneumococcus*)
Neonates	Group B strep, *Klebsiella, E. coli*
Children	*H. influenzae, Meningococcus, Pneumococcus*
Adults	Gram-positive cocci, anaerobes, aerobic bacilli

State how each of the following parameters is affected in septic shock:

Temperature	↑ (though 15% present with hypothermia)
Respirations	↑
HR	↑
BP or total peripheral resistance (TPR)	↓
Cardiac output	↑
Pulmonary capillary wedge pressure	↑ (or sometimes normal)

What is the first-line management of septic shock?

Aggressive IV fluids, vasopressors, IV empiric antibiotics, and removal of potential source (eg, catheter, IV line)

Make the Diagnosis

18-y/o student returns to clinic with a rash after being treated with ampicillin for fever and sore throat; PE: tonsillar exudates and enlarged posterior cervical lymph nodes; labs: ↑ lymphocytes and ⊕ heterophil Ab test

Infectious mononucleosis (EBV)

17-y/o swimmer presents with pain and discharge from the left ear; PE: movement of tragus is extremely painful.

Otitis externa

2-m/o with maternal h/o rash and flu in first trimester presents with failure to attain milestones; PE: microcephaly, cataracts, jaundice, continuous machinery-like murmur at left upper sternal border (LUSB), and hepatosplenomegaly (HSM)

Congenital rubella

8-y/o from Connecticut presents with fever, rash, headache, and joint pain after playing in the woods; PE: distinctive macule with surrounding 6-cm target-shaped lesion

Lyme disease

Newborn with h/o intrauterine growth retardation (IUGR) presents with rash and maternal h/o "flu" during first trimester; PE: petechial rash, chorioretinitis, microcephaly, ↓ hearing, and HSM; CBC: thrombocytopenia; head CT: periventricular calcifications

Congenital CMV

25-y/o West Virginian male presents with fever, headache, myalgia, and a petechial rash that began peripherally but now involves his whole body, even his palms and soles; ⊕ OX19 and OX2 Weil-Felix reaction

Rocky Mountain spotted fever (RMSF)

28-y/o with h/o syphilis treatment (5 h ago) with IM penicillin presents with fever, chills, muscle pain, and headache.

Jarisch-Herxheimer reaction

26-y/o sexually active, native-Caribbean presents with painless, beefy-red ulcers of the genitalia and inguinal swelling; peripheral blood smear: Donovan bodies on Giemsa-stained smear

Granuloma inguinale

31-y/o obese female presents with pruritis in her skin fold beneath her pannus; PE: whitish-curd-like concretions beneath the abdominal pannus; w/u: budding yeast on 10% KOH prep

Cutaneous candidiasis

35-y/o male presents with recurrent Giardia infection and respiratory infections. Labs: ↓ serum IgG

Common variable immunodeficiency aka hypogammaglobulinemia

25-y/o female presents with homogenous white vaginal discharge with fishy odor; PE: no vaginal erythema, vaginal pH >4.5, wet mount: "clue cells"

Bacterial vaginosis

25-y/o female presents with "cottage-cheese," non-odorous vaginal discharge with significant vaginal irritation.

Candidal vaginitis

25-y/o female presents with yellow-green, pruritic, "frothy" vaginal discharge; PE: erythemetous cervix

Trichomonas vaginalis

30-y/o HIV positive man presents with new erythemetous and violaceous macules and large nodules throughout his body.

Kaposi's sarcoma (caused by human herpesvirus 8)

65-y/o man who lives in nursing home presents with headache, lethargy, confusion, nausea, vomiting, diarrhea, and abdominal pain; PE: high fever and relative bradcardia; labs: hyponatremia, ↑ liver enzymes, ↓ phosphate, azotemia, ↑ creatinine kinase

Legionella pneumophila pneumonia

GASTROENTEROLOGY

Diarrhea

Name the four major pathophysiologic mechanisms for chronic diarrhea:	1. Increased secretion 2. Altered intestinal motility 3. Osmotic load 4. Inflammation
What two laboratory tests can be used to distinguish between osmotic and secretory diarrhea?	1. Fasting (persistent diarrhea if secretory) 2. Stool osmotic gap (gap >50 → osmotic diarrhea)

What additional labs are useful in the w/u of osmotic diarrhea?	D-Xylose test, Schilling test (terminal ileum), lactose challenge, and pancreatic enzymes
What is the main cause of surreptitious diarrhea?	Mg^{2+} laxative overuse
Which syndrome is characterized by irregular bowel movements, abdominal pain, and comorbid psychiatric disorders (in 50% of cases)?	Irritable bowel syndrome

Name the food poisoning bacteria associated with the following:

Reheated rice	*Bacillus cereus*
Reheated meat dishes	*Clostridium perfringens*
Improperly canned food	*Clostridium botulinum*
Contaminated seafood or raw oysters	*Vibrio parahaemolyticus* and *Vibrio vulnificus*
Meats, mayonnaise, custards	*S. aureus*
Undercooked meats	*E. coli* O157:H7
Raw poultry, milk, eggs, and meat	*Salmonella*

Name six infectious causes of bloody diarrhea:	1. *Salmonella* 2. *Shigella* 3. *Campylobacter jejuni* 4. Enteroinvasive and enterohemorrhagic *E. coli* 5. *Yersinia enterocolitica* 6. *Entamoeba histolytica*

Name the diarrhea-causing organism associated with the following statements:

Most common cause of diarrhea in infants	Rotavirus
10-12 bloody and mucous diarrhea stools per day due to ingestion of cysts	*E. histolytica*
Comma-shaped organisms causing rice-water stools	*Vibrio cholera*
Second to rotavirus as a cause of gastroenteritis in kids	Adenovirus (serotypes 40 and 41)
Bloody diarrhea; very low ID_{50}; nonmotile	*Shigella*
Usually transmitted from pet feces	*Y. enterocolitica*

Motile; lactose nonfermenter; causes bloody diarrhea	*Salmonella*
Comma- or S-shaped organisms causing bloody diarrhea; associated with Guillain-Barré syndrome	*C. jejuni*
Watery diarrhea with extensive fluid loss in AIDS patient	*Cryptosporidium*
Foul-smelling diarrhea after returning from a camping trip	*Giardia lamblia*
Watery diarrhea caused by antibiotic-induced suppression of colonic flora	*Clostridium difficile*
Avoid antibiotic therapy; hemolytic-uremic syndrome (HUS) is a possible complication.	*E. coli* 0157:H7
AIDS	*Cryptosporidium, Mycobacterium avium complex (MAC), Isospora*
Pseudoappendicitis	*Yersinia*

Inflammatory Bowel Disease

Ulcerative colitis (UC) or Crohn's disease?

Pancolitis with crypt abscesses	UC
Fistulas and fissures	Crohn's disease
Associated with ankylosing spondylitis	Both
Associated with sclerosing cholangitis	UC
Amyloidosis	Crohn's disease
Longitudinal ulcers	Crohn's disease
Punched-out aphthous ulcers	Crohn's disease
Can lead to toxic megacolon	UC
Increased risk of colorectal carcinoma	UC >>> Crohn's
Skip lesions	Crohn's disease
Can involve any portion of the GI tract (usually *terminal ileum and colon*)	Crohn's disease

"String sign" on x-ray (due to bowel wall thickening)	Crohn's disease
Associated with pyoderma gangreosum	Both
Transmural inflammation	Crohn's disease
Noncaseating granulomas	Crohn's disease
Cobblestone mucosa	Crohn's disease
Bloody diarrhea	UC
Watery diarrhea	Crohn's disease
Nephrolithiasis	Crohn's disease
Stricture formation	Crohn's disease
Psuedopolyps	UC
Rectal involvement	UC
May mimic acute appendicitis	Crohn's disease

What is the key component of a diagnostic w/u of a patient with suspected inflammatory bowel disease (IBD)?	Colonoscopy with mucosal biopsies
What additional radiologic tests are useful in the w/u of Crohn's disease?	Upper GI series and small bowel follow through
What are the five classes of medical treatment of IBD?	1. Immunosuppressive agents (6-MP, azathioprine, methotrexate, cyclosporine) 2. 5-ASA derivatives (mesalamine, sulfasalazine) 3. Steroids (helpful in acute disease and during exacerbations) 4. Antibiotics (metronidazole for anal disease) 5. Monoclonal antibodies to tumor necrosis factor (TNF)-α (infliximab)
What are the indications for surgery in a patient with Crohn's disease?	1. Intestinal obstruction (most common indication for surgery) 2. Anorectal abscesses 3. Abdominal abscesses (percutaneous drainage) 4. Fistulas 5. Intractable disease

What are the two options for operative management of an obstruction in Crohn's disease?	Bowel resection versus strictureplasty
What complication can occur in a patient with multiple bowel resections?	Short gut syndrome (diarrhea, malabsorption)
Is surgery usually curative for Crohn's disease?	No
What are the indications for surgery in a patient with UC?	1. Uncontrolled hemorrhage 2. Fulminant colitis 3. Toxic megacolon 4. Dysplasia or cancer 5. Intractable disease
What are the three classic signs and symptoms of toxic megacolon?	1. Fever 2. Abdominal pain 3. Acutely distended colon
What is the *initial* treatment of toxic megacolon?	Nothing by mouth (NPO), IV fluids nasogastric (NGT), and antibiotics
What surgical options are commonly used in patients with refractory UC?	Total proctocolectomy, distal rectal mucosectomy, and ileonal pull through
What is the risk of colon cancer in patients with UC?	1%-2% at 10 years; 1% increase in risk every year thereafter
What are the recommendations for colon cancer surveillance in patients with UC?	Yearly colonoscopy after 10 years of disease
Is surgery curative for UC involving the colon?	Yes
What extraintestinal manifestations of UC are cured by surgery?	Pathology of the skin, eyes, and joints
What extraintestinal manifestations of UC are made worse by surgery?	Liver disease

Liver

Name the viral hepatitis agent(s) described by the following statements:	
Fecal-oral transmission	Hepatitis A virus (HAV) and hepatitis E virus (HEV)

Infection leads to a carrier state.	Hepatitis B virus (HBV), hepatitis C virus (HCV), and hepatitis D virus (HDV) delta agent **Note:** 80% of patients with HCV and 10% with HBV will develop chronic hepatitis.
Defective virus requiring hepatitis B surface antigen (HBsAg) as its envelope	HDV (delta agent)
Sexual, parenteral, and transplacental transmission	HBV, HCV, HDV
High mortality rate in pregnant women	HEV
Most common cause of hepatitis associated with IV drug use in the United States	HCV
Long incubation (~3 months)	HBV
Increased risk of hepatocellular carcinoma	HBV, HCV
Immune globulin vaccine available	HAV, HBV (and HDV)
Name the hepatitis serologic marker associated with the following descriptions:	
Antigen found on surface of HBV; continued presence suggests carrier state	HBsAg
Antigen associated with core of HBV	Hepatitis B core antigen (HBcAg)
Antigen in the HBV core that indicates transmissibility	Hepatitis Be antigen (HBeAg)
Ab suggesting low HBV transmissibility	Hepatitis Be antibody (HBeAb)
Acts as a marker for HBV infection during the "window" period	Hepatitis B core antibody (HBcAb) (IgM in acute stage)
Provides immunity to HBV	HBsAb
What is the "window" period of a hepatitis infection?	Period during acute infection when HBsAg has become undetectable, but HBsAb has not yet appeared
Name an important indicator of hepatitis B transmissibility:	HBeAg

Name six common causes of cirrhosis:	1. Chronic alcoholism 2. Hereditary hemochromatosis 3. Primary biliary cirrhosis 4. Wilson disease (hepatolenticular degeneration) 5. Viral (HBV, HCV) 6. α_1-Antitrypsin deficiency

List the effects of hepatic failure on the following body systems:

Ocular	Scleral icterus
Dermatologic	Jaundice and spider nevi
Reproductive	Testicular atrophy, gynecomastia, and loss of pubic hair
Hematopoietic	Anemia, bleeding tendency ($\downarrow$ coagulation factors), and pancytopenia
Neurologic	Coma, hepatic encephalopathy (asterixis, hyperreflexia), and behavioral changes
Renal	Hepatorenal syndrome (acute renal failure [ARF] $2°$ to hypoperfusion)
GI	Esophageal varicies, peptic ulcer, and hemorrhoids

Name the liver disorder associated with each of the following findings:

Mallory bodies	Alcoholic hepatitis
Occlusion of IVC or hepatic veins with centrilobular congestion → congestive liver disease; associated with polycythemia, pregnancy, and hepatocellular carcinoma	Budd-Chiari syndrome
Viral infection and salicylates in kids	Reye syndrome
Copper deposition in liver, kidney, brain, and cornea → asterixis, basal ganglia degeneration, and dementia	Wilson disease (hepatolenticular degeneration)
AST:ALT >2	Alcoholic hepatitis
Microvesicular fatty change occurring with fatal childhood hepatoencephalopathy	Reye syndrome

State the etiology of cirrhosis associated with the following clinical or pathologic findings:

Panacinar pulmonary emphysema	α_1-Antitrypsin deficiency
Decreased ceruloplasmin	Wilson disease (hepatolenticular degeneration)
Triad of bronze diabetes, skin pigmentation, and micronodular pigment cirrhosis	Hereditary hemochromatosis
Antimitochondrial antibodies	Primary biliary cirrhosis
Kayser-Fleischer ring	Wilson disease (hepatolenticular degeneration)
Micronodular fatty liver, portal HTN, asterixis, jaundice, and gynecomastia	Chronic alcohol abuse
↑ ferritin, transferrin, and total iron; ↓ total iron-binding capacity (TIBC)	Hereditary hemochromatosis **Note:** total body iron is sometimes high enough to trigger metal detectors.

What test can be used to determine the etiology of ascites?	Paracentesis and serum-ascites albumin gradient (SAAG)
What is the mechanism of disease indicated by a SAAG <1.1 versus >1.1? (SAAG = ascites albumin − serum albumin)	SAAG <1.1: protein leakage SAAG >1.1: imbalance of hydrostatic and oncotic pressure
Name four etiologies of ascites with SAAG <1.1:	1. Malignancy 2. Tuberculosis 3. Pancreatitis 4. Nephrotic syndrome
Name five etiologies of ascites with SAAG >1.1:	1. Cirrhosis 2. Hepatic metastases 3. Budd-Chiari syndrome 4. Cardiac disease 5. Myxedema
What are the four therapeutic options for ascites?	1. Salt restriction 2. Diuretics (spironolactone and furosemide) 3. Large-volume paracentesis 4. Peritoneovenous shunting

Name the three general etiologic categories of portal HTN:

1. *Perisinusoidal* (eg, splenic/portal vein thrombosis, schistosomiasis)
2. *Sinusoidal* (cirrhosis → 90% of all causes)
3. *Postsinusoidal* (eg, right heart failure, hepatic vein thrombosis, constrictive pericarditis)

Name five complications of portal HTN:

1. Ascites
2. Spontaneous bacterial peritonitis (SBP)
3. Hepatorenal syndrome
4. Hepatic encephalopathy
5. Esophageal varices

What must be present in ascitic fluid to make the diagnosis of SBP?

>250 PMNs/mL or >500 WBCs

Name three clinical findings in portal HTN resulting from the portal-systemic collateral circulation:

1. Esophageal varices
2. Caput medusa
3. Hemorrhoids

What is the diagnostic test for bleeding varices?

Esophagogastroduodenoscopy (EGD)

What methods are used to control acute upper GI bleeding caused by bleeding esophageal varices?

Endoscopic sclerotherapy, band ligation, IV vasopressin, and balloon tamponade with Sengstaken-Blakemore tube

What is the main interventional procedure used to manage portal HTN?

Shunt procedure (eg, transjugular intrahepatic portacaval shunt [TIPS])

What is the main complication of a shunt procedure?

Worsening of hepatic encephalopathy (2° to ↓ flow to liver)

What is the classification system used in cirrhosis?

Child's criteria (A, B, or C—worst)

What five criteria are used for classification in the Child's system?

1. Bilirubin
2. Albumin
3. Ascites
4. Encephalopathy
5. Nutrition

Name two drugs used to treat hepatic encephalopathy:

1. Lactulose (↓ ammonia absorption)
2. Neomycin (decreases ammonia production from GI tract)

What is the only definitive therapy for cirrhotic liver disease?

Liver transplant

What are the three absolute contraindications for liver transplantation?	1. Infection outside of hepatobiliary system (eg, AIDS) 2. Metastatic liver disease 3. Uncorrectable coagulopathy

Make the Diagnosis

20-y/o female presents with bloody diarrhea and joint pain; PE: abdominal tenderness, guaiac ⊕ stool; w/u: ↑ ESR and CRP, HLA-B27 ⊕; colonoscopy: granular, friable mucosa with pseudopolyps throughout the colon

Ulcerative colitis

28-y/o patient with h/o of UC presents with severe abdominal pain, distention, and high fever; PE: severe abdominal tenderness; w/u: leukocytosis; abdominal x-ray (AXR): dilated (>6 cm) transverse colon

Toxic megacolon

A cirrhotic patient presents with massive hematemesis; PE: jaundice, ↓ BP, ↑ HR, ascites; w/u: pancytopenia, ↑ ALT and AST; EGD: actively bleeding vessel with numerous cherry red spots

Esophageal varices

38-y/o male with recent h/o fatigue, excessive thirst, and impotence presents with hyperpigmentation of his skin; PE: cardiomegaly, HSM; w/u: ↑ glucose, ferritin, transferrin, and serum iron

Hemochromatosis (hereditary)

19-y/o female with recent h/o behavioral disturbance presents with jaundice and resting tremor; PE: pigmented granules in cornea and HSM; w/u: ↓ serum ceruloplasmin

Wilson disease

29-y/o with h/o intermittent jaundice since receiving blood transfusion after motor vehicle accident (MVA) 2 years ago; PE: right upper quadrant (RUQ) tenderness, hepatomegaly; w/u: negative HBV serology

Chronic hepatitis C (HCV) infection

31-y/o female presents with 10-month h/o foul-smelling, greasy diarrhea; PE: pallor, hyperkeratosis, multiple ecchymoses, and abdominal distention; w/u: abnormal D-xylose test

Celiac disease

A patient with recent h/o antibiotic use for sinus infection presents with fever, bloody diarrhea, and abdominal pain; PE: tender abdominal examination, guaiac positive stool; w/u: leukocytosis; colonoscopy: tan nodules seen attached to erythematous bowel wall with superficial erosions

Pseudomembranous colitis (*C. difficile* colitis)

60-y/o white male presents with steatorrhea, weight loss, arthritis, and fever; w/u: small bowel biopsy shows PAS-positive macrophages and gram-positive bacilli.

Whipple disease

A patient presents with sudden onset of severe watery diarrhea, vomiting, and abdominal discomfort 4 h after eating potato salad at a picnic; the symptoms resolve spontaneously within 24 h.

S. aureus-induced diarrhea

23-y/o female with h/o depression presents with abdominal discomfort and irregular bowel habits; w/u: stool cultures, electrolytes, and imaging studies all WNL

Irritable bowel syndrome

A patient traveling in Mexico presents with bloody diarrhea, vomiting, and abdominal cramps 16 h after drinking tap water; PE: low-grade fever, abdominal pain; w/u: ova and parasites in stool

Entamoeba histolytica—induced diarrhea

19-y/o Jewish female with h/o chronic abdominal pain presents with recurrent UTIs and pneumaturia; PE: diffuse abdominal pain; CT: enterovesical fistula; colonoscopy: skip lesions of linear ulcers and transverse fissures giving cobble-stone appearance to mucosa

Crohn's disease

28-y/o homosexual male presents with RUQ pain, fever, anorexia, N/V, dark urine, and clay-colored stool; PE: jaundice, tender hepatomegaly; w/u: ↑↑ AST/ALT, ↑ bilirubin/ALP, normal WBC

Acute viral hepatitis

54-y/o male with h/o HCV presents with increased abdominal girth, jaundice, and altered mental status; PE: asterixis, scleral icterus, hemorrhoids, bilateral lower extremity edema, ascites, and caput medusae; w/u: pancytopenia, ↑AST/ALT/ALP/bilirubin; US: nodular liver

Portal hypertension/cirrhosis

26-y/o female presents with pale, foul-smelling, bulky stools associated with abdominal pain and bloating occurring after meals; PE: normal; w/u: fecal WBC/RBC WNL, ↑osmotic gap, fecal fat WNL

Lactose intolerance

28-y/o male with h/o Crohn disease (s/p surgical resection) presents with increased diarrhea, steatorrhea, and abdominal pain; PE: weight loss; w/u: fecal WBC/RBC WNL, ↑ osmotic gap, ↑ fecal fat, Schillings test abnormal

Malabsorption (short gut syndrome)

RENAL/GENITOURINARY

Basic Metabolism and Electrolytes

How is the anion gap calculated?	$Na^+ - (Cl^- + HCO_3^-)$
What is a normal anion gap?	8-12 mEq/L
List six causes of nongap metabolic acidosis:	1. Diarrhea 2. Renal tubular acidosis (RTA) 3. Spironolactone 4. Total parenteral nutrition (TPN) 5. Glue sniffing 6. Hyperchloremia
List nine possible causes of anion gap metabolic acidosis:	"MUD PILERS" 1. **M**ethanol 2. **U**remia 3. **D**iabetic ketoacidosis (DKA) 4. **P**araldehyde 5. **I**NH or **I**ron tablet overdose 6. **L**actic acidosis 7. **E**thylene glycol or **E**thanol 8. **R**habdomyolysis (massive) 9. **S**alicylate toxicity
List the most common mechanism of respiratory acidosis:	Hypoventilation; causes include lung obstruction (acute/chronic lung disease) and neuromuscular disorders (sedatives, weakening of respiratory muscles)
List four causes of respiratory alkalosis:	1. Hyperventilation (2° to hypoxia) 2. Early ASA ingestion 3. Pregnancy 4. Cirrhosis
List four causes of chloride-responsive (*dry*) metabolic alkalosis:	1. Excessive vomiting 2. Villous adenoma 3. Diuretics 4. Contraction alkalosis

List three diseases causing chloride-unresponsive (*wet*) metabolic alkalosis:

1. Cushing syndrome
2. Conn syndrome
3. Bartter syndrome

Ingestion of what substance can cause both a metabolic acidosis and respiratory alkalosis?

ASA (salicylates)

Name the primary acid/base disturbance and the compensatory response that has occurred in the following:

pH >7.4, P_{CO_2} >40 mm Hg

Metabolic alkalosis → hypoventilation

pH <7.4, P_{CO_2} >40 mm Hg

Respiratory acidosis → renal HCO_3^- reabsorption

pH >7.4, P_{CO_2} <40 mm Hg

Respiratory alkalosis → renal HCO_3^- secretion

pH <7.4, P_{CO_2} <40 mm Hg

Metabolic acidosis → hyperventilation

Name the electrolyte imbalance associated with the following conditions:

Diabetes insipidus (DI), dehydration, and osmotic diuresis

Hypernatremia

ARF, adrenal insufficiency, spironolactone, rhabdomyolysis, acidosis, insulin deficiency, and digitalis poisoning

Hyperkalemia

Syndrome of inappropriate secretion of antidiuretic hormone (SIADH), volume depletion, water intoxication, cirrhosis, heart failure, and hyperglycemia

Hyponatremia

Diarrhea, alkalosis, hypomagnesemia, laxative abuse, RTA, vomiting, and Bartter syndrome

Hypokalemia

Acute pancreatitis, hypomagnesemia, post-parathyroidectomy (most common cause)

Hypocalcemia

Hyperparathyroidism and malignancy (eg, multiple myeloma, breast cancer, and squamous cell cancers)

Hypercalcemia

Malnutrition, alcoholism, DKA, and pregnancy

Hypomagnesemia

Name the ECG changes associated with the following electrolyte imbalances:

Hyperkalemia

In order:
1. Peaked T waves
2. ↑ PR interval
3. Loss of P wave
4. Widened QRS complex
5. Sine wave

Hypokalemia

T-wave flattening, U waves, ST depression, and AV block

Hypocalcemia

↑ QT interval

Hypomagnesemia

Torsade de pointes

Name the main causes of hypercalcemia:

"CHIMPANZEES"

Calcium supplementation

Hyperparathyroidism (most common)

Iatrogenic/Immobility

Milk-alkali syndrome

Paget disease

Neoplasm (very common)

Zollinger-Ellison (ZE) syndrome

Excess vitamin A

Excess vitamin D

Sarcoidosis (or other granulomatous disease)

Provide the treatment for the following electrolyte disturbances:

Hypernatremia

Isotonic NS or LR (correct over a 48-72 h period)

Hyponatremia

If *Na$^+$ <120* → hypertonic NS; if *hypovolemic* → isotonic NS (**Note:** rapid ↑ in plasma Na$^+$→ **central pontine myelinolysis**); if *euvolemic or hypervolemic* → salt and water restriction

Hyperkalemia

"See big K die" → "C BIG Kay Di"

Calcium gluconate (stabilizes cardiac membrane)

Bicarbonate

Insulin and **G**lucose

Kayexalate

Diuretics (loop) and **D**ialysis

Hypercalcemia	IV hydration, loop diuretic (**"loops lose calcium"**), bisphosphonates (especially when caused by malignancy) **Note:** avoid thiazide diuretics.
Hypokalemia	PO supplements, IV infusion of <10 mEq/h, K^+-sparing diuretics
What electrolyte imbalance can result in hypokalemia refractory to supplementation?	Hypomagnesemia
What lab abnormality may cause serum calcium to be falsely low?	Hypoalbuminemia
Name the two classic PE findings associated with hypocalcemia:	1. Chvostek's sign (facial spasm elicited from tapping the facial nerve) 2. Trousseau's sign (carpal spasm after arterial occlusion with BP cuff)

Name the type of RTA associated with each of the following:

Decreased bicarbonate reabsorption	Type II (proximal)
Aldosterone deficiency or resistence	Type IV
Decreased H^+ excretion; nephrocalcinosis	Type I (distal)
Hyperkalemia	Type IV
Most common RTA	Type IV
Fanconi syndrome	Type II (proximal)
Hyporeninemic hypoaldosteronism	Type IV
Seen commonly in diabetes mellitus	Type IV

Renal Failure

What are the three etiologies of ARF?	1. Prerenal (hypoperfusion) 2. Intrinsic (renal) 3. Postrenal (obstructive); can evaluate cause with renal US
Name five causes of prerenal ARF:	1. Hypovolemia 2. Heart failure 3. Sepsis 4. Burns 5. ↓ Renal blood flow (RBF) (eg, ↓CO, renal artery stenosis)

Name five causes of intrinsic ARF:	1. Acute tubular necrosis (ATN) 2. Acute interstitial nephritis 3. GN 4. Autoimmune vasculitis 5. Renal ischemia (eg, thromboembolism)
Name four causes of postrenal ARF:	1. Prostate disease 2. Nephrolithiasis 3. Pelvic tumors 4. Recent pelvic surgery
How is FE_{Na} (fractional excretion of sodium) calculated?	$(Urine_{Na+}/plasma_{Na+})/(urine_{Cr}/plasma_{Cr})$

Which type of ARF is associated with the following findings?

$FE_{Na} <1\%$	Prerenal
$FE_{Na} >4\%$	Postrenal
Hyaline urine casts	Prerenal
Muddy brown/granular casts	Intrinsic (ATN)
BUN:Cr >20	Prerenal
Red cell casts	Intrinsic (GN)
White cell cast ± eosinophils	Intrinsic (allergic nephritis)
Enlarged prostate	Postrenal
⊕ ANCA	Intrinsic (vasculitis)
Urine osmolality >500	Prerenal
White cells, while cell casts	Postrenal (pyelonephritis)

Name three types of insults to the proximal tubules that result in ATN:	1. Ischemia 2. Direct toxins (contrast dye, ampho B, aminoglycosides) 3. Myoglobinuria/hemoglobinuria
What two classes of drugs most commonly cause interstitial nephritis?	1. Penicillins 2. Nonsteroidal anti-inflammatory drugs (NSAIDs)
What unique UA finding is associated with drug-induced interstitial nephritis?	Eosinophilia
What lab value is used to diagnose and follow renal failure?	Creatinine

List the effects of uremia on the following systems:

Nervous system	Asterixis, confusion, seizures, and coma
Cardiovascular system	Fibrinous pericarditis
Hematologic system	Anemia and immunosupression coagulopathy
GI system	Nausea, vomiting, and gastritis
Dermatologic system	Pruritis, and uremic frost (urea crystals on skin) in severe uremia
Endocrine system	Glucose intolerance

List six nonuremic complications of ARF:

1. Metabolic acidosis
2. Hyperkalemia → arrhythmias
3. Na^+ and H_2O excess → pulmonary edema and CHF
4. Hypocalcemia → osteodystrophy (from failure to secrete active vitamin D)
5. Anemia (↓ erythropoietin [EPO] secretion)
6. HTN (from renin hypersecretion)

What are the indications for dialysis treatment?

"AEIOUY"

Acidosis (unresponsive)

Electrolyte abnormality (hyperkalemia)

Ingestion of toxins (salicylates, barbiturates, lithium, ethylene glycol)

Overload (fluid)

Uremic symptoms (pericarditis, encephalopathy)

Y-not?

Infections

What type of infection presents with flank pain, costovertebral angle tenderness, fever, dysuria, pyuria, and bacteriuria?

Acute pyelonephritis

What are the two major causes of pylonephritis?

1. Ascending infection
2. Hematogenous seeding

What are the most common organisms responsible for acute pyelonephritis?

E. coli > *Proteus* > *Enterobacter* (same as UTIs)

What is the greatest risk factor for pyelonephritis?	Vesicoureteric reflux (or incompetency)
All children <7 y/o presenting with their first UTI should undergo what radiologic test to screen for reflux?	Voiding cystourethrogram
List three possible sequelae of acute pyelonephritis:	1. Abscess 2. Renal papillary necrosis 3. Renal scars
What condition is characterized by broad renal scarring, loss of renal parenchyma over time, and thyroidization of kidneys?	Chronic pyelonephritis
Which renal disease presents with multiple 3-4-cm cysts in bilaterally enlarged kidneys resulting in chronic renal failure in adults?	Autosomal-dominant (adult) polycystic kidney disease (ADPKD); 50% have end-stage renal disease (ESRD) by age 60
What are the two most common presenting symptoms of ADPKD?	1. Pain 2. Hematuria
What may the abdominal examination reveal in ADPKD?	Large palpable kidney
Name five other findings associated with ADPKD:	1. Cerebrovascular aneurysm (berry aneurysm) 2. HTN 3. Nephrolithiasis 4. Mitral valve prolapse 5. Hepatic cysts
What is the prognosis for autosomal-recessive polycystic kidney disease (PKD)?	Death in the first few years of life

Glomerular Disease

What syndrome is characterized by hematuria, ARF, HTN, and mild proteinuria?	Nephritic syndrome
What syndrome is characterized by massive proteinuria (>3.5 g/d), generalized edema, hyperlipidemia, and hypoalbuminemia?	Nephrotic syndrome

Classify each of the following
statements as characteristics of
nephrotic or nephritic syndrome:

Increased risk of infections	Nephrotic
Gross hematuria, oliguria	Nephritic
Anticoagulation therapy is indicated to reduce risk of DVT and renal vein thrombosis.	Nephrotic
"Foamy urine"	Nephrotic
Transient oliguria usually followed by spontaneous diuresis	Nephritic
Hyperlipidemia, lipiduria	Nephrotic
Dyspnea and ascites	Nephrotic (severe edema)
One-third of cases associated with systemic diseases (lupus, diabetes, or amyloidosis)	Nephrotic
Smoky brown urine with RBC casts	Nephrtic

Name the glomerulopathy most closely
associated with the following findings:

Apple-green birefringence under polarized light	Renal amyloidosis
GN with lens dislocation, nerve deafness, and posterior cataracts	Alport syndrome
Nodular glomerulosclerosis, glomerular capillary basement membrane thickening	Diabetic glomerulosclerosis (Kimmelstiel-Wilson disease)
Young African American males	Focal-segmental glomerulonephritis (FSGN)
c-ANCA	Wegener's granulomatosis
Most common cause of nephrotic syndrome in children	Minimal change disease (lipoid nephrosis)
Most common cause of ESRD in the United States	Diabetic glomerulosclerosis
Commonly associated with HIV infection, heroin addiction, sickle cell disease, and obesity	FSGN
Mesangial widening and recurrent hematuria and proteinuria	IgA nephropathy (Berger disease)
Associated with hepatitis C	Membranoproliferative glomerulonephritis (MPGN)

Responds well to steroids	Minimal change disease (aka steroid responsive nephropathy)
Responds to plasma exchange and pulsed steroids	Goodpasture syndrome
X-linked recessive defect in α_5 chain of collagen type IV (COLA4A5)	Alport syndrome
Asymptomatic familial hematuria	Thin membrane disease (glomerular basement membrane [GBM] is only 50%-60% of normal thickness)
"Wire loop lesions"	SLE—lupus nephropathy, diffuse proliferative pattern
Upper-respiratory granulomatous inflammation ($\rightarrow$ hemoptysis) and kidney with necrotizing vasculitis	Wegener's granulomatosis
Increased ASO titer	Postinfectious GN
Most common glomerulopathy worldwide	IgA nephropathy (Berger disease)
Pulmonary hemorrhage and hemosiderin-filled macrophages in sputum	Goodpasture syndrome
Associated with URI or GI infections, $\uparrow$ in kids	IgA nephropathy (Berger disease)
Associated with hepatitis B infection	Membranous GN
Antiglomerular basement membrane antibodies	Goodpasture syndrome
Antinuclear antibody (ANA) $\oplus$	SLE
Immunofluorescence $\rightarrow$"lumpy-bumpy" granular IgG or C3 deposits	Postinfectious GN
Immunofluorescence $\rightarrow$ smooth, linear IgG deposits	Goodpasture disease (crescentic GN)
Immunofluorescence $\rightarrow$ "spike and dome"	Membranous GN
Immunofluorescence $\rightarrow$ "tram-track," double-layered basement membrane	Membranoproliferative nephropathy
GN associated with $\downarrow$ complement levels (3)	SLE, MPGN, postinfectious GN
Associated with multiple myeloma or chronic inflammatory disease	Renal amyloidosis
Light microscopy appears normal; electron microscopy shows fusion of epithelial foot processes.	Minimal change disease

Give the treatment for each of the following glomerulopathies:

FSGN	Supportive (protein and salt restriction, diuretic therapy, antihyperlipidemics) and prednisone
Postinfectious GN	Supportive (prognosis very good)
Wegener granulomatosis	High-dose steroids and cytotoxic agents
IgA nephropathy	Steroids for flares (20% progress to ESRD)
SLE	Steroids, and cyclophosphamide (for advanced types)

Renal Calculi

Name the type of renal calculus associated with each of the following findings:

1° hyperparathyroidism	Calcium phosphate
Idiopathic hypercalciuria	Calcium oxalate
Radiolucent stones	Uric acid
Staghorn calculi	Struvite ($MgNH_4PO_4$)
Hexagonal crystals	Cystine
Associated with *Proteus, Pseudomonas, Providencia,* and *Klebsiella* UTIs	Struvite ($MgNH_4PO_4$)
Forms in acidic urine (pH <5.5)	Uric acid
Amino acid transport defect	Cystine
Goat, myeloproliferative disease, or chemotherapy	Uric acid
Crohn's disease	Calcium oxalate
Xanthine oxidase deficiency	Uric acid
~ 80% of renal stones	Calcium oxalate/calcium phosphate

Name eight risk factors for nephrolithiasis:

1. ↓ fluid intake
2. Hypercalcemia
3. Gout
4. Enzyme deficiency
5. RTA
6. Medications (allopurinol, chemotherapy, loop diuretics)
7. Inflammatory bowel disease
8. ⊕ FH

What is the typical presentation of nephrolithiasis?	Acute onset of **severe**, colicky flank pain radiating to the groin with N/V and hematuria
Name three tests to evaluate for nephrolithiasis:	1. UA (hematuria, pH, crystals under microscope) 2. Abnormal XR (90% of stones are radiopaque) 3. Helical CT scan without contrast (now **the test of choice**)
What is the initial treatment for calculi?	Hydration and analgesia
What antihypertensive ↓ [Ca^{2+}] in urine?	Thiazide diuretic
Stones up to what size can pass spontaneously?	Typically <5 mm
What is the treatment for stones >5 mm but <3 cm?	Extracorporeal shock wave lithotripsy (ESWL)

Urinary Tract

What is the differential diagnosis of hematuria?	"S2I3T3" Stricture Stones Infection Inflammation Infarction Tumor Trauma TB
What is the most common malignant tumor of the urinary tract?	Bladder (transitional cell) cancer (↑ in males >60 y/o)
What is the strongest risk factor for urinary tract malignancies?	**Smoking** (also chronic infections, aniline dye, calculi)
What is the most common presenting symptom of bladder cancer?	Painless, gross hematuria
What is the diagnostic test of choice?	Cystoscopy with biopsy
What is the etiology of squamous cell bladder cancers? (rare)	*Schistosoma haematobium*

Name four treatment options for bladder cancer:	1. Intravesical chemotherapy 2. Transurethral resection 3. Surgery ± radiation 4. Chemotherapy alone
What is the classic triad of renal cell carcinoma?	1. Hematuria 2. Flank pain 3. A Palpable mass
Name five risk factors of renal cell carcinoma:	1. Male gender 2. Smoking 3. Obesity 4. Acquired cystic kidney disease in ESRD 5. von Hippel-Lindau disease

Prostate

What is the most common cause of cancer in men?	Prostate cancer (lung cancer is the leading causes of cancer **death** in men, followed by prostate cancer)
What digital rectal examination (DRE) finding suggests prostate cancer?	Firm nodules
What is the histologic type of >95% of prostate cancers?	Adenocarcinoma
What percentage of patients with prostate cancer present with metastatic disease?	40% (most are initially asymptomatic)
What is the most common site of metastasis for prostate cancer?	Bone (vertebrae); must rule out in any elderly male with back pain
Why do obstructive symptoms occur less frequently than in BPH?	Cancer usually begins in the peripheral zone while BPH occurs in the central zone.
What serum marker is used to detect and follow prostate cancer?	Prostate-specific antigen (PSA) >4 ng/mL
Name four causes of an elevated PSA other than carcinoma:	1. BPH 2. Prostatitis 3. UTI 4. Prostatic trauma
How is prostate cancer definitively diagnosed?	Transrectal biopsy of suspicious lesions

Name an alternative to prostatectomy for treatment of localized prostate cancer:	Radiation therapy
Name the two most common complications of prostatectomy:	1. Impotence 2. Incontinence
List three treatment options for metastatic disease:	Androgen ablation via: 1. Luteinizing hormone-releasing hormone (LHRH) agonists (leuprolide) 2. Antiantrogens (flutamide) 3. Orchiectomy
What are the screening recommendations for prostate cancer?	DRE and PSA every year for patients >50 y/o (or patients >40 y/o if African American or ⊕ FH)
What are the two types of symptoms that result from BPH?	1. **Obstructive** (hesitancy, weak stream, incomplete emptying, urinary retention) 2. **Irritative** (nocturia, ↑ frequency, urge incontinence, opening hematuria)
What may be found on PE in a patient with BPH?	Diffusely enlarged prostate with a rubbery texture
Is PSA helpful in monitoring BPH?	No (useful in posttreatment cancer patients)
Name four complications of BPH:	1. Bladder outlet obstruction 2. Urinary stasis (leading to infections and calculi) 3. Chronic urinary retention and overflow 4. Renal failure
What lab value can help detect obstructive uropathy?	Creatinine level (elevated if obstructive lesion)
What medical options are used to treat BPH?	5-α-Reductase inhibitors (finasteride) and α-receptor blockers (terazosin)
What are the indications for surgery in BPH?	Symptomatic obstruction: 1. Postvoid residual volume >100 mL 2. Multiple bouts of gross hematuria 3. Recurrent UTIs
Name the most common surgical procedure for BPH:	Transurethral resection of the prostate (TURP)

Erectile Dysfunction

Name the two categories of erectile dysfunction (ED):	1. **Primary:** never been able to have sustained erections 2. **Secondary:** acquired
Name three causes of primary ED:	1. Psychologic 2. Gonadal ($\downarrow$ testosterone) 3. Endocrine (thyroid, Cushing, etc)
Name three causes of 2° ED:	1. Drug-induced (tricyclic antidepressants [TCAs], diuretics, antipsychotics) 2. Vascular disease (eg, veno-occlusive dysfunction) 3. Neurologic disease
What is one finding that can make the distinction between psychologic and organic ED?	Nocturnal or early-morning erections
Provide four treatment options for ED:	1. Sildenafil (or other PDE5 inhibitors) 2. Intracavernosal prostaglandins 3. Vacuum-constriction device 4. Penile prosthesis
What drug is an absolute contraindication for patients taking sildenafil?	Nitrates (combined effects of lowering BP → myocardial ischemia)

Testes

Name the testicular disorder associated with the following statements:

Failure of descent of testicle before 1 y/o; $\uparrow$ risk of cancer	Cryptorchidism
Malignant testicular tumor that is highly radiosensitive	**Sem**inomas = **Sen**sitive to radiation
Worst prognosis of all testicular tumors; highly invasive; elevated β-hCG levels	Choriocarcinoma
Slow growing tumor usually discovered and removed before metastasis; most common type of testicular cancer	Seminomas (type of germ cell tumor)

Associated with an abnormally high attachment of the tunica vaginalis around the distal end of the spermatic cord (*bell clapper deformity*)	Testicular torsion (usually bilateral)
Usually presents as a firm, painless mass	All testicular tumors
Rapid onset of testicular pain, swelling, and absence of flow on Doppler ultrasound	Testicular torsion (testicle unsalvageable after 6 h)
Bag of worms on testicular examination	Varicocele
α-Fetoprotein (AFP) is often elevated in this form of testicular cancer.	Endodermal sinus tumor
Treatment of cryptorchidism	Orchiopexy after age 1 but before 5 (to preserve fertility); orchiectomy later in life to avoid risk of testicular cancer

Make the Diagnosis

25-y/o-Asian male presents with N/V, and colicky right flank pain; PE: acute distress and costovertebral angle (CVA) tenderness; w/u: hematuria and discrete radiopacities on abdominal XR

Renal stones

45-y/o with documented h/o aortic atheromatous plaques presents with recent onset, severe left flank pain, and hematuria; abd CT: wedge-shaped lesion in the left kidney

Renal infarct

55-y/o with long h/o DM presents with increasing fatigue and edema; PE: ↑ BP, retinopathy, and pitting edema; w/u: severe proteinuria and glycosuria

Diabetic nephropathy (glomerulosclerosis)

21-y/o sexually active female presents with frequency and dysuria; PE: afebrile, suprapubic tenderness, no CVA tenderness; w/u: *E. coli* ⊕ urine cultures

UTI

25-y/o male presents with hemoptysis, dark urine, and fatigue; PE: bilateral crackles at lung bases; w/u: oliguria, hematuria, and anti-GBM Abs

Goodpasture syndrome

7-y/o presents in stupor after ingesting antifreeze; PE: Kussmaul respirations and mental status changes; w/u: anion gap of 21 mEq/L

Metabolic acidosis (ethylene glycol toxicity)

6-y/o boy presents with hematuria and worsening vision; PE: corneal abnormalities, retinopathy, sensorineural hearing loss; w/u: hematuria with dysmorphic red cells

Alport syndrome

3-y/o boy with h/o recent URI presents with facial edema; PE: ascitic fluid in abdomen and pedal edema; w/u: 4+ proteinuria and ↓ serum albumin

Minimal change disease

70-y/o male recently started on an ACE inhibitor presents with weakness, N/V, and palpitations; PE: areflexia; ECG: tall, peaked T waves and wide QRS complex

Hyperkalemia

65-y/o patient with h/o small cell lung cancer presents with lethargy, confusion, and seizures; w/u: serum Na^+ <135 mEq/L, urinary Na^+ >20 mEq/L, and urine osmolality >100 mOsm/kg

SIADH (hyponatremia)

A patient s/p parathyroidectomy presents with muscle cramps, dyspnea, and tetanic contraction; PE: facial spasm with tapping over facial nerve, carpal spasm with arterial occlusion by BP cuff; ECG: ↑ QT interval

Hypocalcemia

A patient on a loop diuretic for CHF presents with muscle weakness, fatigue, and ileus; PE: hyporeflexia,bradycardia; ECG: T-wave flattening, ST depression, and U waves

Hypokalemia

A patient hospitalized for CHF recently started on an aminoglycoside for a UTI develops oliguria, N/V, and malaise; PE: ↑ BP and asterixis; w/u: ↑ Cr, K^+; UA: "muddy brown" casts, FE_{Na+} >3%

ARF (drug-induced ATN)

70-y/o-black male with h/o of lifelong DM presents with peripheral edema, SOB, and oliguria; PE: auscultatory rales, pitting edema, myoclonus, and uremic frost; serum electrolytes: ↑ Cr, hyperkalemia, hypocalcemia, hyperphosphatemia

Chronic renal failure

A female presents with fever, chills, and flank pain; PE: CVA tenderness; UA: leukocyte esterase ⊕, 30 WBC/hpf

Pyelonephritis

32-y/o male presents with pain and hematuria; PE: ↑ BP, palpable kidney, and midsystolic ejection click; abd US: multiple cysts of renal parenchyma; cerebral angiogram: unruptured berry aneurysm

Polycystic kidney disease

12-y/o male with h/o sore throat 2 weeks ago presents with low urine output and dark urine; PE: periorbital edema; w/u: hematuria, ↑ BUN and Cr, ↑ ASO titer

Poststreptococcal GN

45-y/o-Asian male with h/o hepatitis B presents with malaise, edema, and foamy urine; PE: anasarca; w/u: proteinuria (>3.5 g/d), hyperlipidemia, and hypoalbuminemia

Membranous GN

80-y/o male presents with urinary hesitancy, nocturia, and weak urinary stream; PE: diffusely enlarged rubbery prostate; w/u: ↑ Cr, ↑ PSA ; UA is within normal limits (WNL).

Benign prostatic hyperplasia (BPH)

68-y/o-male smoker presents with flank pain and hematuria; PE: fever, palpable kidney mass; w/u: hypercalcemia, polycythemia

Renal cell carcinoma

20-y/o male presents with acute onset of left testicular pain and N/V; PE: swollen, tender testicular in transverse position, absent cremasteric reflex on left side; Doppler: no flow detected in left testicle

Testicular torsion

85-y/o male presents with back pain, weight loss, and weak urinary stream; PE: palpable firm nodule on DRE; w/u: ↑ PSA (5 ng/mL)

Prostate cancer

65-y/o male smoker presents with painless gross hematuria and frequency; PE: obese; UA: hematuria,dysplastic cells; intravenous pyelogram (IVP): bladder filling defect

Bladder cancer (transitional cell carcinoma)

41-y/o male with h/o HTN recently started on β-blocker presents with impotence that started 2 months ago. Reports no early-morning erections; PE: normal size testes and normal lower extremity sensation; w/u: testosterone/prolactin WNL

Drug-induced erectile dysfunction (ED)

22-y/o male with h/o cryptorchism presents with painless enlargement of L testes; PE: L scrotal swelling and a palpable mass; w/u: ↑ AFP

Testicular cancer (endodermal sinus tumor)

16-y/o male with recent h/o gastroenteritis 2 days ago presents with episodic brown urine; PE: unremarkable; w/u: hematuria, mild proteinuria, normal C3

IgA nephropathy

33-y/o male presents with fever, hemoptysis, and hematuria; PE: weight loss and bilateral crackles at lung bases; w/u: hematuria, ⊕ c-ANCA; CXR: bilateral cavitary lesions

Wegener granulomatosis

A patient hospitalized and started on methicillin develops fever, arthralgias, and a pruritic rash; PE: ↑ BP, edema, and diffuse erythematous rash; w/u: oliguria, ↑Cr; UA: eosinophils, WBCs

Allergic interstitial nephritis

65-y/o male with multiple myeloma presents with lethargy and bone pain; PE: altered mental status; ECG: ↓ QT interval

Hypercalcemia

ENDOCRINE

Pituitary

Name the pituitary disorder associated with each of the following:

Most common functional pituitary adenoma	Prolactinoma (adenoma)
Deficiency of gonadotropin-releasing hormone (GnRH) → no 2° sexual characteristics; associated with anosmia	Kallmann syndrome
Polyuria, polydipsia, hypernatremia; associated with tumor, infection, and autoimmune disease	Central/neurogenic DI
Hypopituitarism from postpartum pituitary necrosis	Sheehan syndrome

Enlargement of jaw, hands, feet, and coarsening facial features 2° to ↑ serum growth hormones (GH)	Acromegaly
Pituitary hypersecretion of ADH → hyponatremia, ↓ urine output, mental status changes	SIADH

What are the two general ways pituitary masses can present clinically?

1. Mass effects (bitemporal hemianopsia, CN palsies)
2. Endocrine effects (amenorrhea, galactorrhea, hyperthyroidism, ↓ libido)

What is the treatment of choice for symptomatic nonfunctional pituitary adenomas?

Transspheniodal surgical resection

What is the medical treatment of choice for a prolactinoma?

Bromocriptine

What two proteins are used to diagnose acromegaly?

1. GH
2. IGF (insulin-like growth factor)-1 (made in liver in response to GH)

What medical treatment is used to treat acromegaly?

Somatostatin (GH inhibitor)—used if no surgical cure

Patients with acromegaly are at increased risk for what type of malignancy?

Colonic polyps (close screening with colonoscopy is indicated)

Name the two subtypes of DI and describe the mechanism of disease:

1. Central DI: posterior pituitary fails to secrete ADH.
2. Nephrogenic DI: kidneys fail to respond to ADH.

What are some common presenting symptoms in a patient with DI?

Polydipsia, polyuria, and persistent thirst with dilute urine

What is the relationship between urine osmolality and serum osmolality in DI?

Low urine osmolality with high serum osmolality

How are psychogenic polydipsia and DI differentiated using a water deprivation test?

DI patients continue to produce a high volume of dilute urine while psychogenic polydipsia patients will no longer produce urine.

What is the radiologic test of choice to detect pituitary abnormalities?

Magnetic resonance imaging (MRI) (better soft-tissue resolution)

Which hormone level remains normal in panhypopituitarism?	Prolactin (under chronic inhibition by dopamine secreted by the hypothalamus)
Which hormones need to be replaced in panhypopituitarism?	Cortisol, levothyroxine, and estrogen or testosterone
Name five etiologies of SIADH:	1. CNS (head trauma, subarachnoid hemorrhage, tumor, hydrocephalus) 2. Pulmonary (small cell lung CA, sarcoidosis, pneumonia, abscess) 3. Endocrine (Conn syndrome, hypothyroidism) 4. Drugs (antipsychotics, antidepressants, oral hypoglycemics) 5. Surgery (intracranial, intrathoracic)
How is the diagnosis of SIADH made?	Urine osmolality >50-100 mOsm/kg (hyperosmolar urine) with current serum hyposmolarity, and urinary sodium >20 mEq/L
What is the treatment for SIADH?	Fluid restriction and hypertonic saline (acutely); demeclocycline (chronic)
What is the treatment of DI?	Central DI: DDAVP (desmopressin—an ADH analog) Nephrogenic DI: salt restriction and ↑ water intake

Thyroid

Name four lab findings in hyperthyroidism:	1. ↓ Thyroid-stimulating hormone (TSH) (in 1°) 2. ↑ free T4 3. ↑ total T4 4. ↑ T3 uptake
Name four lab findings in hypOthyroidism:	1. ↑ TSH (very sensitive for 1°) 2. ↓ free T4 3. ↓ total T4 4. ↓ T3 uptake
Describe how each of the following organ systems are affected by (1) hypothyroidism (HypO) and (2) hyperthyroidism:	
Metabolism	**HypO:** hypometabolic state, cold intolerance **Hyper:** ↑ basal metabolic rate (BMR), heat intolerance

Cardiac	**HypO:** exercise intolerance, $\downarrow$ HR, shortness of breath, pericardial effusion
	Hyper: $\uparrow$ CO, $\uparrow$ HR, palpitations, cardiomegaly (long-term)
Ocular	**HypO:** periorbital myxedema
	Hyper: staring gaze, lid lag; Graves $\rightarrow$ exophthalmos
Neuromuscular	**HypO:** hypoactive deep tendon reflexes (DTR)
	Hyper: $\uparrow$ sympathetic activity, fine tremor, hyperactive reflexes
Skin	**HypO:** coarse, dry skin; hair loss
	Hyper: warm, moist, and flushed skin; fine hair; Graves $\rightarrow$ pretibial myxedema
GI	**HypO:** weight gain, constipation
	Hyper: weight loss despite hyperphagia, $\uparrow$ GI motility
Other	**HypO:** menorrhagia, $\downarrow$ pitch of voice, depression
	Hyper: menstrual abnormalities, osteoporosis, anxiety, insomnia
Name three possible treatments for hyperthyroidism:	1. Propranolol (control symptoms) followed by radioablation 2. Antithyroid drugs (methimazole, propylthrouvnel [PTU]) 3. Thyroidectomy
What is the most common long-term side effect of radioablation or thyroidectomy?	HypOthyroidism
What is the treatment of choice for hypOthyroidism?	Levothyroxine
What feared complication of hyperthyroidism can be induced by an infection or surgery?	Thyroid storm (tachycardia, **high-output cardiac failure**, and coma)
What is the mortality rate of thyroid storm?	25%
What is the treatment of thyroid storm?	1. β-blockers 2. PTU 3. Iodine 4. Steroids

Name the thyroid disorder associated
with each of the following statements:

Child with coarse facial features, short stature, mental retardation, and umbilical hernia	Congenital hypothyroidism (cretinism)
Goiter occurring with high frequency in iodine-deficient areas	Endemic goiter
Painless enlargement of thyroid of autoimmune etiology; requires long-term treatment with levothyroxine	Hashimoto's thyroiditis
Triad of diffuse thyroid hyperplasia, ophthalmopathy, and dermopathy	Graves disease
Postviral, painful inflammation of thyroid; usually self-limited, treated with ASA or corticosteroids	Subacute (granulomatous, de Quervain) thyroiditis
Painless goiter that can occur postpartum; can cause hypothyroidism	Subacute lymphocytic (painless) thyroiditis
Thyroid-stimulating immunoglobulin (TSI), a TSH-receptor Ab, stimulates thyroid hormone production	Graves disease
Extreme thyroid enlargement (>2 kg) causing mass effects; most patients are euthyroid; may require surgical debulking	Multinodular goiter
Antimicrosomal Ab, antithyroglobulin Ab	Hashimoto's thyroiditis
Most common thyroid carcinoma	Papillary carcinoma
Calcitonin-secreting tumor associated with multiple endocrine neoplasia (MEN) syndromes	Medullary carcinoma
Carcinoma presenting as a single nodule with uniform follicles	Follicular carcinoma
Aggressive carcinoma of older patients with pleomophic cells; dismal prognosis	Anaplastic (undifferentiated) carcinoma
Which two types of thyroid cancer have the worst prognosis?	1. Medullary 2. Anaplastic
What is the test of choice for the detection of metastases from thyroid malignancies?	Radioactive iodine scan

What is the treatment for a malignant thyroid nodule?	Surgical resection
Are most thyroid nodules benign or malignant?	Benign
What findings are associated with ↑ risk of thyroid cancer?	1. Prior neck radiation 2. **Cold** nodule 3. Firm, fixed, rapidly growing solitary nodule 4. Hoarseness/dysphagia
What is the diagnostic test of choice to evaluate a thyroid nodule?	Fine needle aspiration (FNA)

Name the MEN syndrome associated with the following descriptions:

Pheochromocytoma, thyroid medullary carcinoma, and parathyroid adenomas	MEN 2 (Sipple syndrome)
Tumors of the pituitary, pancreatic islet cells, and parathyroids	MEN 1 (Wermer syndrome)
Tumors in MEN2 plus tall, thin habitus, prominent lips, and ganglioneuromas of the tongue and eyelids	MEN 3 (MEN 2b)
AD inheritance	All MEN syndromes

Parathyroid

Name the parathyroid disorder associated with each of the following statements:

Caused by chronic renal failure or ↓ vitamin D	2° hyperparathyroidism
Most commonly due to parathyroid adenomas (90%)	1° hyperparathyroidism
Etiologies include congenital gland absence, postsurgical, and autoimmune destruction	HypOparathyroidism
Caused by an autonomous hormone secreting adenoma	3° hyperparathyroidism
Autosomal recessive (AR) end-organ resistance to PTH → short stature and short third/fourth metacarpals	Pseudohypoparathyroidism

What four systems are primarily affected by hyperparathyroidism?

"Painful bones, renal stones, abdominal groans, and psychic moans"
1. **Painful bones:** osteitis fibrosa cystica, osteoporosis, fractures
2. **Renal stones:** nephrolithiasis, nephrocalcinosis
3. **Abdominal groans:** constipation, peptic ulcer disease (PUD), pancreatitis, N/V
4. **Psychic moans:** depression, lethargy, seizures

What is the treatment of chronic symptomatic hypercalcemia from hyperparathyroidism?

Parathyroidectomy with preoperative bisphosphonates

Name two postoperative complications of parathyroidectomy:

1. Recurrent laryngeal nerve injury (hoarseness)
2. HypOcalcemia

Adrenals and Steroids

Name the four etiologies for hypercortisolism:

1. Exogenous glucocorticoids (most common overall)
2. Pituitary ACTH hypersecretion (eg, adenoma)
3. Hypersecretion of cortisol (eg, adrenal hyperplasia)
4. Ectopic ACTH (eg, small cell lung cancer)

What is the most common cause of endogenous hypercortisolism?

Cushing **disease** (1° pituitary adenoma)

Name eight classic clinical findings of Cushing syndrome:

1. Hyperglycemia/hypokalemia/HTN
2. Virilization and menstrual disorder in women
3. Moon facies
4. Truncal obesity
5. Buffalo hump
6. Skin changes (thinning, purple striae)
7. Osteoporosis: vertebral compression fractures
8. Immune suppression-susceptibility to infection

What two tests are used to screen for Cushing syndrome?

1. Overnight low-dose dexamethasone suppression test
2. 24-h urine-free cortisol

What test is used to localize the source of hypercortisolism?

1. Check ACTH levels ($\uparrow$ = ectopic/pituitary; $\downarrow$ = adrenal)
2. High-dose dexamethasone suppression test (when ACTH $\uparrow$, suppression suggests pituitary disease)

Name the adrenal disorder associated with each of the following statements:

Aldosterone-secreting adenoma causing HTN, hypokalemic, hypernatremia, and metabolic alkalosis

Conn syndrome
(1° hyperaldosteronism)

21-hydroxylase deficiency (autosomal recessive) → cortisol deficiency and $\uparrow$ adrenal andorgens

Congenital adrenal hyperplasia

Endotoxin-mediated massive adrenal hemorrhage

Waterhouse-Friderichsen syndrome (caused by *Neisseria meningitidis*)

Deficiency of aldosterone and cortisol occurs 2° to adrenal atrophy or autoimmune destruction; may cause hypotension

1° chronic adrenocortical insufficiency (Addison disease)

Hypothalamic-pituitary axis (HPA) disturbance (eg, abrupt cessation of glucocorticoid treatment) causing failure of ACTH secretion

2° adrenocortical insufficiency

Bilateral hyperplasia of zona glomerulosa caused by stimulation of renin-angiotensin-aldosterone (RAA) system

2° hyperaldosteronism

Results from rapid steroid withdrawal or sudden $\uparrow$ in glucocorticoid requirements

1° acute adrenocortical insufficiency (adrenal crisis)

Chromaffin cell tumor usually in adults; results in episodic hyperadrenergic symptoms

Pheochromocytoma

Malignant, small, round, blue cell tumor of medulla in kids associated with N-*myc* oncogene amplification

Neuroblastoma

How is 1° and 2° adrenocortical insufficiency differentiated?

2° is not associated with hyperpigmentation.

What substance can be measured to differentiate between 1° and 2° hyperaldosteronism?

Renin ($\uparrow$ in 2° hyperaldosteronism)

What is the drug of choice for hyperaldosteronism?	Spironolactone (aldosterone antagonist)
What is the "rule of 10s" for pheochromocytomas?	10% malignant 10% bilateral 10% extraadrenal 10% kids 10% familial 10% calcify
What are the five Ps of pheochromocytoma (symptoms)?	Pressure, Pain (headache), Perspiration, Palpitations, and Pallor
What substances are secreted from pheochromocytomas and how are they detected?	Epinephrine and norepinephrine; diagnosed by ↑ urinary secretion of catecholamines and their metabolites (metanephrine, VMA, etc)
What is the treatment of a pheochromocytoma?	Surgical resection (preoperative α- and β-blockade)
Why is it necessary to block α-receptors before giving a β-blocker?	To prevent unopposed vasoconstriction
What are the electrolyte and CBC abnormalities in Addison disease?	Hyponatremia, hyperkalemia, and eosinophilia
What test is used to evaluate the etiology of Addison disease?	ACTH stimulation test (↑ ACTH and ↓ cortisol = Addison; ↓ ACTH and ↑ cortisol = 2° cause)
What is the treatment of adrenal insufficiency?	Replacement of glucocorticoids and mineral corticoids
What must be administered to a patient with Addison disease during periods of stress (eg, surgery, trauma, or infection)?	Stress-dose steroids
What are the two main etiologies of 1° hyperaldosteronism and their respective treatments?	Adrenal adenoma (Conn syndrome) → adrenalectomy; bilateral hyperplasia → spironolactone

Pancreas-Diabetes Mellitus

What endocrine disease should be suspected in a patient who presents with poor wound healing or recurrent vaginal candidiasis?	Diabetes mellitus (DM)

Describe the classic acute presentation of type 1 diabetes mellitus:	Polydipsia, polyuria, polyphagia, weight loss, and DKA if extreme
What is the proposed mechanism of islet cell destruction in type 1 DM?	Environmental triggering of autoimmunity to islet β-cells
What is the theorized cause of type 2 DM?	Obesity increases insulin resistance and causes β-cell dysfunction.
Name three criteria to diagnose DM:	1. Fasting glucose >126 mg/dL 2. Random glucose >200 mg/dL with symptoms 3. 2-hr glucose >200 mg/dL during 75-g oral glucose tolerance test (on two separate occasions)
What is HbA_{1c} and what is it used for?	Percent of glycosylated hemoglobin in blood; used to measure diabetic control over last 90-120 days (average lifespan of RBC)-goal <7%
Name the acute complication of DM associated with the following descriptions:	
Abdominal pain, vomiting, Kussmaul respirations, fruity/acetone breath odor, anion gap metabolic acidosis, and mental status changes usually precipitated by stress (infection, drugs, MI, or noncompliance with insulin therapy)	DKA—type 1 DM
Profound dehydration, extreme hyperglycemia (>600 mg/dL), mental status changes without acidosis	Hyperosmolar hyperglycemic nonketotic coma (HHNK)—type 2 DM
What are the three major components of the treatment of DKA?	1. Fluids (add dextrose when glucose falls below 200 mg/dL) 2. Insulin 3. Potassium
Why must K^+ be replaced in a patient with DKA even though serum levels are usually elevated?	Acidosis and insulonopenia force K^+ out of cells initially but the total body potassium levels may be low.
What is the mortality rate of HHNK?	50%
What is the main treatment of HHNK?	Aggressive fluid replacement and insulin

Describe the effect(s) of long-term DM on each of the following organ systems:

Cardiovascular (macrovascular) — Atherosclerosis → CVA, MI, PVD

Urinary (microvascular) — Glomerular (glomerulosclerosis, proteinuria); vascular (arteriosclerosis → HTN, CRF); infectious (UTIs, pyelonephritis, necrotizing papillitis)

Nervous (microvascular) — Motor and sensory peripheral neuropathy, autonomic degeneration/dysfunction (orthostatic hypotension)

Eye (microvascular) — Retinopathy, cataract formation, blindness

Skin — Xanthomas, abscesses from ↑ infections and poor wound healing, fungal infections

What two factors are shown to correlate with the severity of microvascular complications?

1. Glycemic control
2. Duration of disease

What preventive measures must be taken to minimize complications of DM?

1. Annual dilated retinal examination
2. Microalbuminuria yearly with spot microalbumin/Cr ratio, goal <30 mg/g
3. Annual podiatrist examination
4. BP control (<130/80)
5. Lipid control (LDL<100, TGs <150, HDL >40)
6. HbA_{1c} every 3-6 months (<7%)

Name the appropriate therapy for each of the following clinical scenarios in a diabetic:

Proliferative retinopathy — Laser photocoagulation

Microalbuminuria — ACE inhibitor or ARB

Neuropathy — Gabapentin and amitriptyline

Type 1 diabetes — Insulin

Newly diagnosed type 2 diabetes refractory to lifestyle modifications — Oral hypoglycemics

Type 2 diabetes refractory to monotherapy with an oral hypoglycemic agent — Oral hypoglycemic agent with a different mechanism or begin insulin therapy

For each of the following types of
insulin, state the onset, peak, and
duration of action:

Insulin lispro

Onset: 5-10 m; peak: 60-90 min;
duration: 2-4 h

NPH or Lente insulin

Onset: 2 h; peak: 4-8 h; duration:
12-18 h

Ultralente insulin

Onset: 3-5 h; peak: 10-16 h; duration:
12-20 h

Insulin glargine

Onset: 2 h; peak: none (peakless);
duration >24 h

For each oral hypoglycemic, state
the mechanism and unique toxicity
of each:

Biguanides (eg, metformin)

↓ hepatic gluconeogenesis and ↑
peripheral uptake of glucose; risk
of lactic acidosis; contraindicated
in the elderly and in pts with renal
disease

Sulfonylureas (eg, glyburide,
glipizide, glimepiride)

↑ insulin secretion; may cause
hypoglycemia and weight gain

Thiazolidinediones (eg, pioglitazone,
rosiglitazone)

↑ peripheral insulin responsiveness;
may cause weight gain, edema, and
hepatotoxicity

α-Glucosidase inhibitors (eg,
acarbose, miglitol)

↑ GI absorption of carbohydrates; may
cause GI upset/flatulence

Name four causes of 2° diabetes
mellitus:

1. Pancreatic disease (eg,
   hemochromatosis, pancreatitis,
   pancreatic carcinoma)
2. Pregnancy (gestational diabetes)
3. Cushing syndrome
4. Other endocrine disorders (eg,
   acromegaly, glucagonoma,
   hyperthyroidism)

Name the criteria to diagnose
metabolic syndrome:

Must meet three of the following
criteria:
1. Abdominal obesity
2. TG ≥150 mg/dL
3. HDL <40 in men and <50 in
   women
4. BP ≥130/85 mm Hg or taking
   antihypertensive meds
5. Fasting glucose ≥110 mg/dL

Name the following complications
of diabetic management:

Nocturnal hypoglycemia causing elevated morning glucose 2° to release of counterregulatory hormones	Somogyi effect
Abrupt early-morning hyperglycemia caused by reduced effectiveness of insulin	Dawn phenomenon

Name the islet cell tumor associated
with each of the following statements:

Most common is let cell tumor	Insulinoma (β-cell tumor)
2° diabetes mellitus, necrolytic migratory erythema	Glucagonoma (α-cell tumor)
Associated with ZE syndrome	Gastrinoma
Associated with WDHA (watery diarrhea, hypokalemia, and achlorhydria) syndrome	VIPoma
2° diabetes mellitus, cholelithiasis, steatorrhea	Somatostatinoma (δ-cell tumor)
Clinically characterized by Whipple's triad	Insulinoma (β-cell tumor)

Name the clinical findings of Whipple's triad:	1. Hypoglycemia 2. Concurrent CNS dysfunction 3. Reversal of CNS symptoms with glucose
What is ZE syndrome?	Hypersecretion of gastric HCl, recurrent PUD, and hypergastinemia (associated with MEN)
How is ZE syndrome diagnosed?	↑ serum gastin level with secretin stimulation test

Make the Diagnosis

31-y/o presents with loss of libido, galactorrhea, and irregular menses; PE: bitemporal hemianopsia; w/u: negative β-hCG

Prolactinoma

Patient taking lithium presents to clinic with polyuria and polydipsia; w/u: urine specific gravity <1.005, urine osmolality <200 mOsm/kg, hypernatremia

Diabetes insipidus (DI)

30-y/o white female presents with weight loss, tremor, and palpitations; PE: brisk DTR, ophthalmopathy, pretibial myxedema; w/u: ↓ TSH, ↑ T4, ↑ T3 index

Graves disease

40-y/o female presents with fatigue, constipation, and weight loss; PE: puffy face, cold dry hands, coarse hair, and enlargement of thyroid gland; w/u: ↑ TSH, ↓ T3 and T4, ⊕ antimicrosomal Ab and antithyroglobulin Ab

Hashimoto disease

32-y/o female with h/o recurrent PUD presents with episodes of hypocalcemia and nephrolithiasis; w/u: fasting hypoglycemia, ↑ gastrin levels, and hypercalcemia

MEN 1

70-y/o presents with episodal HTN, nephrolithiasis, and diarrhea; PE: ↑ BP, thyroid nodule; w/u: ↑ calcitonin levels, ↑ urinary catecholamines

MEN 2

A female patient presents with bone pain, kidney stones, depression, and recurrent ulcers; w/u: hypercalcemia, hypophosphatemia, and hypercalciuria

Hyperparathyroidism

35-y/o female presents with weight gain, irregular menses, and HTN; PE: ↑ BP, weight in face and upper back, hirsutism, multiple ecchymoses; w/u: ↑ ACTH levels and suppression with high-dose dexamethasone suppression test

Cushing disease

45-y/o with recent h/o coarsening of facial features presents with headaches and states that his shoes no longer fit; PE: enlarged jaw, tongue, hands, and feet, and bitemporal hemianopia; w/u: ↑ IGF-1

Acromegaly

9-y/o female presents with muscle cramps; PE: rounded face with flat nasal bridge, abnormal dentition, positive Trousseau's sign and Chvostek's sign, and shortened metacarpals

Albright hereditary osteodystrophy (pseudohypoparathyroidism)

50-y/o female presents with HTN, muscle weakness, and fatigue; w/u: hypokalemia, hypernatremia, and metabolic alkalosis

Conn syndrome

30-y/o female presents with progressive weakness, weight loss, and N/V; PE: hyperpigmentation of skin, ↓ BP; w/u: hyperkalemia, hyponatremia, and eosinophilia

Addison disease

40-y/o presents with episodes of HA, diaphoresis, palpitations, and tremor; PE: ↑ BP, ↑ HR; w/u: ↑ in urinary VMA and homovanillic acid

Pheochromocytoma

17-y/o white female with h/o DM presents with diffuse abdominal pain, N/V, and slight confusion; PE: ↓ BP, shallow rapid breathing pattern; w/u: ↑ glucose (300 mg/dL), hypokalemia, hypophosphatemia, and metabolic acidosis

DKA-DM type I

60-y/o diabetic obese patient found at home confused and disoriented; PE: ↓ BP, ↑ HR; w/u: glucose >1000, pH is WNL

HHNK-DM type II

50-y/o female presents with h/o weakness, blurred vision, and confusion several hours after meals, which improves with eating; w/u: ↑ fasting levels of insulin and hypoglycemia

Insulinoma

78-y/o male presents with rapidly growing palpable thyroid mass and associated hoarseness; PE: firm, fixed, nontender nodule, anterior cervical lymphadenopathy; FNA: "Orphan Annie" nuclei and psammoma bodies

Papillary thyroid carcinoma

21-y/o female presents with increased amounts of dark facial hair, acne, and menstrual abnormalities; PE: ↑BP, hirsutism; w/u: ↑androgens and cortisol precursors (ie, progesterone)

Congenital adrenal hyperplasia (21-hydroxylase deficiency)

26-y/o male presents with tender thyroid, malaise, runny nose, and cough; PE: fever, tender thyroid but no palpable mass, cervical adenopathy; w/u: ↓ uptake on radioactive iodine uptake (RAIU)

Subacute (de Quervain's) thyroiditis

54-y/o female with h/o uncontrolled DM-type 2 presents for regular follow-up visit; PE: obese, ↑BP (165/90); w/u: ↑TG (230), ↓HDL(40), ↑HbA$_{1c}$ (8.2)

Metabolic syndrome

55-y/o female with rheumatoid arthritis presents with confusion, abdominal pain, and N/V after abruptly stopping prednisone treatment; PE: altered mental status, fever, ↑ HR, ↓BP, no skin hyperpigmentation; w/u: normal K$^+$, hyponatremia, eosinophilia, ↓ cortisol

Adrenal crisis (2° adrenal insufficiency)

HEMATOLOGY/ONCOLOGY

Anemias

What are some common presenting symptoms in an anemic patient:	Fatigue, DOE, angina, headache, dizziness, and syncope
List five of the most common causes of microcytic anemia:	1. Iron deficiency 2. Lead poisoning 3. Chronic disease (sometimes normocytic) 4. Sideroblastic 5. Thalassemia
List four of the most common causes of normocytic anemia:	1. Sickle cell 2. Aplastic 3. Acute blood loss 4. Hemolytic anemia
List five of the most common causes of macrocytic anemia:	1. Liver disease 2. Vitamin B_{12} deficiency 3. Folate deficiency 4. Alcoholism 5. Hypothyroidism
What is the primary site of iron absorption?	Duodenum
What are the two most common causes of iron deficiency anemia in adults?	1. Menorrhagia 2. GI blood loss
What is the mechanism of ischemic necrosis of the bones, lungs, liver, brain, spleen, or penis in sickle cell disease?	$\downarrow O_2$ tension $\rightarrow$ abnormal RBCs sickle $\rightarrow$ microvascular occlusions
What two common enzyme deficiencies can cause hemolytic anemia?	1. Glucose-6-phosphate dehydrogenase 2. Pyruvate kinase deficiency
What two autoimmune conditions of the GI tract can cause megaloblastic anemia?	1. Pernicious anemia (due to lack of intrinsic factor [IF] production) 2. Crohn's disease (due to lack of IF-B_{12} complex reabsorption in distal ileum)
How does gastric resection cause megaloblastic anemia?	Parietal cells, which are responsible for IF production may be removed when the gastric fundus is resected.

Name the type(s) of anemia associated with the following clinical or pathologic features:

Abnormal Schilling test	Pernicious anemia
Angular chelitis, koilonychia, pica	Iron deficiency anemia
Autosplenectomy	Sickle cell anemia
Basophilic stipling of erythrocytes, blue/gray discoloration at gumline, wrist/foot drop	Microcytic anemia (lead poisoning)
Celiac sprue	Megaloblastic (folate deficiency) and iron deficiency anemias
Chronic atrophic gastritis	Pernicious anemia
Colon cancer	Iron deficiency anemia (early) and anemia of chronic disease (late)
Crescent-shaped erythrocytes and Howell-Jolly bodies	Sickle cell anemia
↓ Serum iron, normal iron-binding protein saturation, ↓ ferritin, ↓ TIBC	Anemia of chronic disease
↓ Ferritin, ↑ red blood cell distribution width (RDW), ↑ TIBC, ↓ Serum iron, ↓ iron-binding protein saturation	Iron deficiency anemia
↑ Serum iron, maximal iron-binding protein saturation, ↓ ferritin, normal TIBC	Iron overload/hereditary hemochromatosis
Deficiency of α- or β-globin gene synthesis	Thalassemia
Deficiency of decay accelerating factor	Paroxysmal nocturnal hemoglobinuria
Demyelination of the dorsal and lateral tracts of the spinal cord	Pernicious anemia
Diphyllobothrium latum (fish tapeworm) and *G. lamblia* infection	Macrocytic anemia (B_{12} deficiency)
↑ reticulocyte count, indirect hyperbilirubinemia, ↑ LDH, and negative direct Coombs test	Hemolytic anemia
End-stage liver disease	Macrocytic anemia
Oxidative stress on erythrocytes in a G6PD-deficient patient	Hemolytic anemia
"Fishmouth vertebrae" on radiograph	Sickle cell anemia

Gastric carcinoma	Pernicious anemia
Glossitis and peripheral neuropathy	Pernicious anemia
Helmet cells, burr cells, triangular cells	Microangiopathic anemia (2° to disseminated intravascular coagulation [DIC], TTP-HUS), or mechanical heart valves)
Persistently elevated creatinine	Anemia of chronic renal failure
High reticulocyte count	Hemolytic anemia (or acute hemorrhage)
Hypersegmented PMNs	Vitamin B_{12} or folate deficiency anemia
Hypothyroidism	Macrocytic anemia
Leukemias and lymphomas	Autoimmune hemolytic anemia
Fatigue, jaundice, dark urine after consumption of fava beans	Hemolytic anemia (due to G6PD deficiency)
Pancytopenia and fatty infiltration of bone marrow	Aplastic anemia
Malaria or babesiosis	Hemolytic anemia
May be caused by Crohn's disease of the terminal ileum	Macrocytic anemia (B_{12} deficiency)
Microcytosis, atrophic glossitis, esophageal webs (Plummer-Vinson triad)	Iron deficiency anemia (long standing)
Most common type of anemia	Iron deficiency anemia
M. pneumoniae infection	Cold autoimmune hemolytic anemia
NSAIDs, chloramphenicol use	Aplastic anemia
Penicillin, cephalosporin, or quinidine use	Autoimmune hemolytic anemia
AD deficiency of spectrin, positive osmotic fragility test	Hereditary spherocytosis
Priapism	Sickle cell anemia
SLE, chronic lymphocytic leukemia (CLL), lymphomas, drugs; ⊕ direct Coombs test (due to IgG autoantibodies)	Warm autoimmune hemolytic anemia
Reduced erythropoietin	Anemia of chronic disease
Ringed sideroblasts	Sideroblastic anemia
Schistocytes	Microhemangiopathic anemia
Susceptibility to infection by encapsulated organisms	Sickle cell anemia (due to functional asplenia)

Target cells	**"HALT"** Hemolysis Asplenia Liver disease Thalassemia
Unconjugated bilirubinemia, ↑ urine urobilinogen, ↓ hemoglobin, hemoglobinuria, ↓ haptoglobin, hemosiderosis	Hemolytic anemia

Name the type of thalassemia responsible for each of the following findings:

β-Thalassemia associated with growth retardation, frontal bossing and HSM (from extramedullary hematopoesis), jaundice, and iron overload (2° to transfusions), and ↑ Hgb F	β-Thalassemia major (β–/β–) **Note:** β-thalassemia minor (β+/β–) typically asymptomatic
α-Thalassemia associated with mild microcytic anemia, usually asymptomatic	α-Thalassemia minor (two alleles affected) **Note:** when only one allele involved (carrier state) → no anemia
α-Thalassemia associated with pallor, splenomegaly, chronic hemolytic anemia, and intraerythrocytic inclusions	Hgb H disease (three alleles affected)
α-Thalassemia associated with stillborn fetus	Hydrops fetalis (all four alleles affected)

Name three infectious and three noninfectious complications of sickle cell disease:	**Infectious** 1. Osteomyelitis (usually due to *Salmonella*) 2. Pneumococcal and *H. influenzae* pneumonia 3. Parvovirus B_{19} infection causing a plastic anemia **Noninfectious** 1. High-output cardiac failure 2. Splenomegaly (in infants) 3. Vasoocclusive crises
What is the treatment of a vasoocclusive sickle crisis?	Oxygen therapy, IV hydration, analgesia (usually opioids)

What treatment may be used in the setting of severe vasoocclusive crises and chest syndrome with respiratory distress?	Exchange transfusions
What chemotherapeutic agent may decrease the frequency of sickle cell crises?	Hydroxyurea

Coagulation Disorders

Name the coagulation disorder associated with the following clinical features:

Classic triad of thrombocytopenia, hemolytic anemia, and ARF	Hemolytic-uremic syndrome (HUS)
Classic triad of HUS + fever and neurologic changes	TTP Remember: "**FAT RN**": **F**ever, **A**nemia (hemolytic), **T**hrombocytopenia, **R**enal failure, **N**eurologic abnormalities
Commonly follows viral URI in children but may be chronic in adults	Idiopathic thrombocytopenic purpura (ITP)
Commonly occurs in the context of sepsis, major hemorrhage (traumatic or obstetric), or malignancies	DIC
X-linked disorder characterized by hemarthroses and GI bleeding; ↑ PTT, normal PT, platelet count, and bleeding time	Hemophilia
AD disorder characterized by episodes of easy bruising, mucosal and GI bleeding	von Willebrand disease
Treated with Factor VIII	Hemophilia A
Treated with Factor IX	Hemophilia B
Commonly in children; may be caused by *E. coli* O157: H7	HUS
Spontaneous bleeding from surgical wounds and venipuncture sites	DIC
Associated with lymphomas, leukemias, HIV infection, and autoimmune diseases	ITP
IgG antiplatelet antibodies (⊕ Coombs)	ITP

↑ bleeding time, ↓ Factor VIII, normal platelet count, normal PT and PTT	von Willebrand disease
Prolonged PT, PTT, ↑ fibrin split products (D-dimer), ↓ Hct, ↓ platelets	DIC (also known as "consumptive coagulopathy")
Schistocytes, ↑ unconjugated bilirubin, ↑ LDH	TTP
First-line therapy is oral steroids; second line is IV immunoglobulin (IVIG), splenectomy, or chemotherapy (commonly, cyclophosphamide)	ITP
First-line therapy is plasmapheresis or IVIG; splenectomy for refractory cases (fatal if untreated)	TTP
Treatment aimed at underlying disorder; treatment for coagulopathy with platelet transfusion, cryoprecipitate; second line: aminocaproic acid	DIC
Mild disease treated with desmopressin; severe disease treated with Factor VIII concentrate	von Willebrand disease

WBC Neoplasia

Name the general type of lymphoma (Hodgkin's or non-Hodgkin's lymphoma [NHL]) associated with the following clinical and pathologic features:

Reed Sternberg (RS) cells secreting interleukin (IL-5)	Hodgkin disease (HD)
Peak incidence from 20 to 40 years of age, more common in women	NHL
Bimodal age distribution but most common in young men	HD
Constitutional symptoms including fever, night sweats, weight loss	Both
Mediastinal lymphadenopathy, contiguous spread	HD
Systemic adenopathy	NHL
Regional lymphadenopathy	HD

Associated with EBV, HIV infection	HD
Peripheral lymphadenopathy, noncontiguous spread	NHL
Lymphadenopathy may become painful with alcohol consumption	HD
Associated with immunosuppression including AIDS	NHL

Leukemias and Lymphomas

Name the general type of leukemia (acute or chronic) associated with the following clinical and pathologic features:	
Immature blast cells predominate	Acute
Mature cell types predominate	Chronic
Bimodal age distribution	Acute
Rapid onset and quickly progressive disease	Acute
Indolent course	Chronic
Common in middle adulthood	Chronic

| What are the three most common medical complications of end-stage leukemia? | 1. Hemorrhage (due to thrombocytopenia) 2. Infection (due to immunosupression) 3. Anemia (due to involvement of bone marrow) |

Name the specific leukemia associated with each of the following demographics:	
Most common leukemia of childhood, peak age 3-4 years	Acute lymphocytic leukemia (ALL)
Most common leukemia in adults	Acute myelogenous leukemia (AML)
Commonly in males 60 and older	CLL

Name the specific leukemia associated with each of the following findings:	
Very high white cell counts, often >200,000	Chronic myelogenous leukemia (CML)
Isolated lymphocytosis	CLL
TdT positive lymphoblasts	ALL

Large, immature myeloblasts predominate	AML
Smudge cells	CLL
Bone marrow is replaced with myeloblasts.	AML
Philadelphia chromosome t(9:22)	CML
Auer rods	AML
Low leukocytic alkaline phosphatase	CML (as well as paroxysmal nocturnal hematuria)
Associated with fatigue, thrombocytopenia (easy bruising), signs of anemia, frequent infections, leukemia cutis, and DIC	AML
Bone pain, fever, generalized lymphadenopathy, HSM, and signs of CNS spread	ALL
Excellent prognosis if treated early	ALL
May progress to AML	CML
Most responsive to therapy	ALL
Associated with prior exposure to radiation	CML
Peripheral leukocytes containing tartarate resistant acid phosphatase and cytoplasmic projections	Hairy cell leukemia

Myeloproliferative Disorders

Name the four chronic myeloproliferative disorders:	1. Chronic myelogenous leukemia 2. Polycythemia vera 3. Essential thrombocytosis 4. Myelofibrosis with myeloid metaplasia
Name the myeloproliferative disorder associated with each of the following clinical and pathologic findings:	
↑ RBC mass and low/normal erythropoietin	Polycythemia vera
Tear drop deformity of erythrocytes, bone marrow hypercellularity	Myelofibrosis with myeloid metaplasia
Plethoric complexion, pruritus after showering, epistaxis, blurred vision, splenomegaly, and epistaxis	Polycythemia vera

Erythromelalgia (throbbing or burning of hands and feet)	Essential thrombocytosis
Basophilia	Polycythemia vera
Widespread extramedullary hematopoesis with megakaryocytic proliferation in the bone marrow	Myelofibrosis with myeloid metaplasia
Hyperviscosity syndrome	Polycythemia vera and essential thrombocytosis
Peripheral thrombocytosis, bone marrow megakaryocytosis, and splenomegaly	Essential thrombocytosis
Treated with ASA, phlebotomy, and/or hydroxyurea	Polycythemia vera
Treated with platelet exchange (for acute exacerbations), hydroxyurea, and anagrelide	Essential thrombocytosis

Name the plasma cell disorder associated with the following clinical and pathologic findings:

Bone pain, osteopenia, pathologic fractures, and "punched-out" lytic lesions on x-ray	Multiple myeloma
Russel bodies and "plymphocytes" (plasmacytoid lymphocytes)	Waldenstrom macroglobulinemia
Bence-Jones proteinuria	Multiple myeloma and Waldenstrom macroglobulinemia
Small M-spike on plasma electrophoresis in an otherwise healthy patient	Monoclonal gammopathy of undetermined significance (MGUS)
Hypercalcemia; renal insufficiency	Multiple myeloma
Hyperviscosity syndrome	Waldenstrom macroglobulinemia
Large M-spike on plasma electrophoresis	Multiple myeloma and Waldenstrom macroglobulinemia
Primary amyloidosis	Multiple myeloma

Name the disease(s) or condition(s) associated with each of the following peripheral blood smear findings:

Atypical lymphocytes	Infectious mononucleosis
Auer rods	AML (M3 subtype)
Basophilic stippling	Lead poisoning
Burr cells (echinocytes)	Burns and uremia

Heinz bodies	G6PD deficiency
Helmet cells, schistocytes	Microangiopathic hemolytic anemia (DIC, TTP, HUS)
Howell-Jolly bodies	Asplenia (due to trauma or functional asplenia due to sickle cell disease)
Hypersegmented PMN nuclei	Megaloblastic anemia
Lymphocytic cerebriform nuclei	Sézary syndrome
Nucleated erythrocytes	Hemolytic anemia
Rouleau formation	Multiple myeloma and Waldenstrom macroglobulinemia
Smudge cells	CLL
Spherocytes	Hereditary spherocytosis and hemolytic anemia
Spur cells (acanthocytes)	Abetalipoproteinemia, liver disease
Target cells (codocytes)	Thalassemias, iron deficiency anemia, liver disease, and sickle cell anemia
Teardrop cells (dacrocytes)	Myelofibrosis
Toxic granulations in leukocytes	Severe infection

Make the Diagnosis

50-y/o with h/o bone marrow transplant for CML 3 weeks ago presents with severe pruritis, diarrhea, and jaundice; PE: violaceous rash on palms and soles; w/u: ↑ bilirubin, ALT, and AST

　　Graft-versus-host disease

1-y/o Greek child presents with pallor and delayed milestones; PE: pallor, skeletal abnormalities, splenomegaly; peripheral blood smear (PBS): hypochromic microcytic RBCs; target cells, fragmented RBCs; skull XR: "hair-on-end" appearance

　　β-Thalassemia

10-y/o with a h/o recurrent chest pain presents with fever and bilateral leg pain; PE: febrile, multiple leg ulcers; PBS shows sickle-shaped erythrocytes; Hgb electrophoresis shows HgbS band.

　　Sickle cell anemia

60-y/o presents with headache, vertigo, blurry vision, pruritus, joint pain; PE: ↑ BP, plethoric, splenomegaly; w/u: Hct 60, mild leukocytosis, and hyperuricemia

　　Polycythemia vera

4-y/o male with a 1-week h/o fever, pallor, headache, and bone tenderness; PE: fever, HSM, and generalized nontender lymphadenopathy; w/u: PBS reveals absolute lymphocytosis with abundant TdT ⊕ lymphoblasts.

Acute lymphoblastic leukemia

27-y/o presents with 2-month h/o fatigue, oropharyngeal candidiasis, pseudomonal UTI, and epistaxis; PE: numerous petechiae and ecchymoses of skin, gingival mucosal bleeding, guaiac ⊕ stools; w/u: ↑ WBCs, PBS shows >30% myeloblasts with Auer rods.

Acute myelocytic leukemia

17-y/o male presents with a 2-month h/o fever, night sweats, and weight loss; PE: nontender, cervical lymphadenopathy, and HSM; CBC: leukocytosis; CXR: bilateral hilar adenopathy; lymph node biopsy: Reed-Sternberg cells

Hodgkin disease

60-y/o male presents with fatigue and anorexia; PE: generalized lymphadenopathy and HSM; CBC: WBC: 250,000, ⊕ direct Coombs test; PBS: small, round lymphocytes predominate with occasional smudge cells.

Chronic lymphocytic leukemia

10-y/o Black child presents with a 3-week h/o a rapidly enlarging, painless mandibular mass; CBC: mild anemia and leukopenia; cytogenetics reveal a t(8:14) translocation; excisional biopsy: "starry-sky" pattern

Burkitt lymphoma

35-y/o presents with a 3-year h/o mild weight loss, anorexia presents with worsening DOE; PE: splenomegaly; CBC: mild anemia, WBC: 125,000; PBS: granulocytosis with <10% myeloblasts; cytogenetics reveal a t(9:22) translocation.

Chronic myelocytic leukemia

55-y/o with a recent h/o streptococcal pneumonia presents with bone pain and weight loss; w/u: mild anemia, hypercalcemia; PBS: rouleau formation; UA: Bence-Jones proteinuria; serum electrophoresis: M-spike; XR: cranial "punched-out" lesions

Multiple myeloma

18-y/o female develops dyspnea and declining mental status 1 hour after a C-section complicated by excess blood loss; PE: mucosal bleeding, large clot in the vaginal vault; coags: ↑ PT and PTT, ↓ platelets, ↑ fibrin split products

Disseminated intravascular coagulation (DIC)

7-y/o with h/o viral URI 1 week ago presents with epistaxis; PE: petechial hemorrhages of nasal mucosa and extremities; w/u: ↓ platelets, normal PT and PTT; bone marrow biopsy: ↑↑ megakaryocytes

Idiopathic thrombocytopenia purpura (ITP)

8-y/o with a h/o vomiting and diarrhea after eating a hamburger last week presents with fatigue, periorbital edema, and oliguria; PE: purpuric rash; CBC: ↓ platelets; PBS: burr cells, helmet cells; UA: RBC casts, proteinuria, hematuria

Hemolytic-uremic syndrome (HUS)

8-y/o with a h/o environmental allergies presents with a painful rash on the legs, abdominal discomfort, joint pain; UA: hematuria and RBC casts; renal biopsy: glomerular mesangial IgA deposits

Henoch-Schönlein purpura

65-y/o female w/ fever and forgetfulness; labs: thrombocytopenia, anemia, shistocytes, ↑ LDH, elevated creatinine

Thrombotic thrombocytopenic purpura (Tx: plasma exchange)

8-y/o male presents with a swollen painful knee; FH: maternal grandfather died from hemorrhage after a cholecystectomy; PE: cutaneous ecchymoses; w/u: gross blood in swollen knee joint, ↑ PTT, normal PT, platelet count, ↑ bleeding time

Hemophilia A

2-y/o male with a h/o recurrent epistaxis presents with the third episode of otitis media in 4 months; PE: eczematous dermatitis; w/u: thrombocytopenia, ↓ IgM, ↑ IgA

Wiskott-Aldrich syndrome

A newborn develops jaundice rapidly during the first day of life; PE: HSM; w/u: severe anemia, ⊕ indirect Coombs test in both mother and newborn

Rh incompatibility

16-y/o female with a h/o menorrhagia presents with fatigue; PE: multiple cutaneous bruises; guaiac ⊕ stools; w/u: ↑ bleeding time, ↓ Factor VIII, normal platelet count, PT and PTT

von Willebrand disease

40-y/o female s/p chest radiation therapy for childhood Hodgkin disease presents with new mass in upper outer quadrant of breast.

Breast cancer

65-y/o male with 100 pack-year hx presents with SOB; PE: JVD, muffled heart sounds; CXR: left lower lobe mass, enlarged cardiac silhouette; TTE: pericardial effusion

Lung cancer metastasis to pericardium (most common breast and lung; also melanoma, uterine cancer, and mesothelioma)

RHEUMATOLOGY/MUSCULOSKELETAL

Spinal Disorders

Name the lower back condition associated with each of the following findings:

Saddle anesthesia with bowel/bladder dysfunction	Cauda equina syndrome
Positive "shopping-cart sign"	Spinal stenosis (patients more comfortable when leaning forward)
Increased pain at night that is unrelieved by positional changes or rest	Malignancy
Positive straight leg raise	Herniated disk → nerve root impingement
Increased pain with rest; pain improves with activity	Ankylosing spondylitis
Paraspinous muscle pain	Back strain (muscle) or sprain (ligamentous)
Pseudoclaudication, ↑ pain with walking	Spinal stenosis
Pain radiating from lower back down to the foot	Sciatica

Name four "red flags" of low back pain:

1. H/o malignancy
2. Constitutional symptoms (fever, weight loss)
3. Bladder/bowel dysfunction
4. Saddle anesthesia

What is the treatment for low back pain in the absence of "red flags"?

Conservative: NSAIDs/acetaminophen, 1-3-day bed rest (85% resolve spontaneously)

What four chronic inflammatory conditions cause fusion of the sacroiliac joints?

The seronegative spondyloarthropathies:
1. ankylosing spondylitis (AS)
2. Reiter syndrome
3. Psoriatic arthritis
4. Enteropathic arthritis

What haplotype is typically associated with >90% of seronegative spondyloarthropathies?

HLA-B27

Joints

What is the definitive diagnostic procedure for acute monoarticular arthritis?	Arthrocentesis
Interpret each of the following arthrocentesis leukocyte counts (cells/mm^3):	
<200 WBCs	Normal joint fluid
<2000 WBCs	Noninflammatory (eg, osteoarthritis [OA])
2000-50,000 WBCs	Mild-to-moderate inflammation (eg, rheumatologic)
50,000-100,000 WBCs	Severe inflammation (eg, septic arthritis or gout)
>100,000 WBCs	Septic joint (until proven otherwise)
What disease is characterized by monoarticular arthritis due to urate crystal deposits?	Gout
What are the two main etiologies of hyperuricemia?	1. Inadequate uric acid *excretion* (most of cases) 2. Uric acid *overproduction* (eg, malignancy, hemolysis, Lesch-Nyhan syndrome)
What is the most common presenting symptom?	Podagra (inflammation of first metatarsophalangeal [MTP] joint)
Why do tophi develop?	Chronic gout → deposits of urate crystals
Name the classic radiographic finding in advanced gout:	Classic "rat-bite" appearance to joint (punched-out erosion with overhanging cortical bone)
What does the joint fluid aspiration of gout reveal?	Needle-shaped, negatively-birefringent crystals under polarized light
What is the treatment for acute gout?	Colchicine and NSAIDs (eg, indomethacin)
What is the maintenance therapy for gout?	**Overproducers** → allopurinol; **underexcreters** → probenecid/sulfinpyrazone (**Note:** continue colchicine because may precipitate acute attack.)

What disease is characterized by calcium pyrophosphate crystal deposition in joints?	Pseudogout
What does the joint fluid aspiration of pseudogout reveal?	Positively-birefringent crystals under polarized light
What chronic, systemic inflammatory arthritis is associated with HLA-DR4 serotype?	Rheumatoid arthritis (RA)

Name the seven diagnostic criteria for rheumatoid authritis (RA):

1. Morning stiffness (>1 hour)
2. Arthritis of three or more joints area (14 possible areas include right or left proximal interphalangeal [PIP], metacarpophalangeal [MCP], wrist, elbow, knee, ankle, and MTP joints)
3. Arthritis of one + hand joints (wrist, MCP, or PIP)
4. Symmetric arthritis
5. Rheumatoid nodules
6. ↑ serum RF—70% of cases
7. Radiographic changes: juxta-articular decalcification and late erosions

Note: 4 of 7 required to classify as RA

What is the term for the classic joint deformity associated with RA?	Boutonniere deformity

Name five extraarticular manifestations of RA:

1. Subcutaneous rheumatoid nodules
2. Asymptomatic pericardial effusions
3. Anemia of chronic disease
4. Nerve entrapment (eg, carpal tunnel syndrome)
5. Pulmonary (effusions, interstitial fibrosis, nodule)

What is the treatment for RA?	**Pain:** first line: NSAIDs, then steroids; **disease-modifying:** first line: hydroxychloroquine, then **methotrexate** (MTX) and biologic agents

Name two of the newer biologic agents used to treat RA:

1. Infliximab (anti-TNF-α Ab)
2. Etanercept (anti-TNF receptor Ab)

What syndrome is characterized by RA, splenomegaly, and leukopenia?	Felty syndrome

Name the seronegative spondylarthropathy associated with the following statements:

Associated with sacroilitis

Ankylosing spondylarthritis

Precipitated by GI or GU infection

Reactive arthritis

Associated with nail pitting and DIP joint involvement

Psoriatic arthritis

Associated with inflammatory bowel disease

Enteropathic arthritis

What special type of reactive arthritis may be seen in HLA-B27 ⊕ males?

Reiter syndrome

How does Reiter syndrome typically present?

"Can't SEE, can't PEE, can't CLIMB UP A TREE" (conjunctivitis, urethritis, and arthritis)

Name two classic dermatologic findings of Reiter syndrome:

1. Keratoderma blennorrhagicum
2. Balanitis circinata

What is the treatment for Reiter syndrome?

Erythromycin (for *Chlamydia*) and NSAIDs for arthritis; may benefit from prolonged tetracycline (3 months)

Osteoarthritis

Name the most common cause of arthritis:

Osteoarthritis (OA)

What noninflammatory arthritis is caused by wear and tear and is relieved by rest?

OA

Name three risk factors for OA:

1. Obesity
2. ⊕ FH
3. H/o joint trauma

Name three classic PE findings in OA:

1. Heberden's nodes (DIP)
2. Bouchard nodes (PIP)
3. Marked crepitus of affected joint

What is the classic radiographic appearance of OA?

Osteophytes and asymmetric joint space loss

What is the management of OA?

Isometric exercise to strengthen muscles at joint; NSAIDs (including cyclooxygenase [COX-2] inhibitors); joint replacement as last resort

Bones

Name the metabolic bone disease associated with each of the following statements:

Osteopenia with normal bone mineralization	Osteoporosis
Results from idiopathic hyperactivity of both osteoblasts and osteoclasts	Paget bone disease (osteitis deformans)
2° to vitamin D deficiency	Rickets (kids), osteomalacia (adults)
Vitamin C deficiency → ↓ osteoid formation	Scurvy
Results from postmenopausal estrogen deficiency, physical inactivity, or calcium deficiency	Osteoporosis
Findings include Harrison groove, pigeon breast, craniotabes, and rachitic rosary	Rickets/osteomalacia
Findings include bleeding gums and "woody leg"	Scurvy
Findings include bone pain, deafness, and high-output cardiac failure	Paget bone disease (osteitis deformans)
Dual energy x-ray absorptiometry (DEXA) scan shows significantly ↓ bone density	Osteoporosis
↑ ALP; sclerotic lesions on XR	Paget bone disease (osteitis deformans)
Death or decay of bone due to local ischemia in the absence of infection	Avascular necrosis (AVN)

Name five risk factors for osteoporosis:	1. Menopause 2. Smoking 3. Low body weight 4. Long-term heparin or glucocorticoid use 5. Alcoholism
What are the treatment options for senile (postmenopausal) osteoporosis?	Most important is prevention; treatment options: estrogen replacement (the only treatment shown to ↑ bone growth), Ca^{2+}, vitamin D, exercise; second line: bisphosphonates and calcitonin

What is the treatment for Paget bone disease?	First line: bisphosphonates; second line: calcitonin
What bone disease is characterized by idiopathic replacement of bone with fibrous tissue?	Fibrous dysplasia
What syndrome is characterized by polyostotic fibrous dysplasia, precocious puberty, and café-au-lait spots?	McCune-Albright syndrome
What pediatric disease is characterized by the triad of skull lesions, DI, and exophthalmos?	Hand-Schüller-Christian disease
What is the most common primary malignant tumor of bone?	Osteosarcoma
Where does osteosarcoma typically occur?	Distal femur and proximal tibia
What is the classic radiographic appearance?	"Sunburst" sign (lytic lesion with spiculated periostitis) and Codman triangle

Fractures and Dislocations

(*See Chap. 2*)

Muscle Diseases

Name the two major categories of muscle diseases:	1. **Neurogenic** (no pain, distal weakness, $\oplus$ fasciculations) 2. **Myopathic** (often painful, proximal weakness, no fasciculations)
Name the specific skeletal muscle disease associated with the following clinical and pathologic findings:	
Anti-ACh receptor antibodies; associated with thymomas and autoimmune disorders	Myasthenia gravis
Most common and most lethal muscular dystrophy	Duchenne's muscular dystrophy
X-linked disease caused by a variety of mutations →↓ functional dystrophin	Becker's muscular dystrophy

Paraneoplastic disorder commonly seen in patients with small cell carcinoma of the lung	Lambert-Eaton syndrome
Decreasing muscle strength with repetitive nerve stimulation	Myasthenia gravis
Muscular disorder associated with gonadal atrophy, baldness, cataracts, cardiomyopathy, and ↓ IgG	Myotonic dystrophy
Antibodies to presynaptic Ca^{2+} channels; ↑ muscle strength with repetitive nerve stimulation	Lambert-Eaton Syndrome
Progressive X-linked disease causing deficiency of dystrophin	Duchenne muscular dystrophy
Variable muscle weakness, most pronounced in occular and facial muscles initially	Myasthenia gravis
Painful, autoinflammatory disorder causing progressive, symmetric muscle weakness, dysphonia, and ↑ serum CPK	Polymyositis
Calf pseudohypertrophy and Gower sign	Duchenne muscular dystrophy
Gait instability (due to weakness of foot dorsiflexion) and involuntary muscle contraction on examination	Myotonic dystrophy

Name the muscle tumor associated with each of the following statements:

Most common tumor in females; estrogen sensitive → may grow during pregnancy and regress during menopause	Leiomyoma
Aggressive, malignant tumor of skeletal muscle; one of the small, round, blue cell tumors of childhood	Rhabdomyosarcoma

Rheumatology

Describe the effect(s) of SLE on each of the following organs:

Skin	Malar rash, discoid rash, photosensitivity
Joints	Arthritis and arthralgia

Central nervous system	Neuropsychiatric changes or seizures (2° to cerebral vasculitis)
Heart	Pericarditis, Libman-Sacks endocarditis (SLE → *LSE*)
Lungs	Pleuritis, pulmonary fibrosis
GI	Oral and nasopharyngeal ulcers
Kidneys	Wire-loop glomerular lesions and mesangial immune complex deposits → glomerulonephritis
Hematology	Hemolytic anemia, leukopenia, thrombocytopenia, Raynaud's phenomena
What pathologic finding is common to all tissues affected by SLE?	Acute necrotizing vasculitis of small arteries and arterioles caused by immune complex deposition
Libman-Sacks endocarditis causes sterile vegetations to form on both sides of which cardiac valve?	Mitral valve
Name five medications capable of inducing a lupus-like syndrome:	1. Hydralazine 2. INH 3. Phenytoin 4. Procainamide 5. Penicillamine
Name the disease related to SLE that is characterized by immune complex deposition at the dermal-epidermal junction:	Discoid lupus erythematosus

Describe the disease associated with the following autoantibodies:

ANA (antinuclear antibodies)	SLE (sensitive but not specific for SLE)
Anti-ACh (acetylcholine)	Myasthenia gravis
Antibasement membrane	Goodpasture disease
Anticentromere	CREST syndrome (**C**alcinosis, **R**aynaud's, **E**sophageal dysmotility, **S**clerodactyly, **T**elangiectasias)
Anti-dsDNA	SLE (highly specific for SLE)
Antiepithelial cell	Pemphigus vulgaris
Antigliadin	Celiac sprue

Antihistone	Drug-induced lupus erythematosus
Anti-IgG Fc	RA (rheumatoid factor [RF])
Anti-Jo1	Myositis
Antimicrosomal	Hashimoto's thyroiditis
Antimitochondrial	Primary biliary cirrhosis
Anti-nRNP (nuclear ribonucleoprotein)	Mixed connective tissue disease
Antiplatelet	ITP
Anti-Scl-70 (DNA topoisomerase 1)	Diffuse scleroderma
Anti-Smith	SLE (highly specific for SLE)
Anti-SS-A (Ro) and anti-SS-B (La)	Sjögren syndrome
Antithyroglobulin	Hashimoto's thyroiditis
Anti-TSHr (TSH receptor)	Graves disease
c-ANCA	Wegener's granulomatosis
Perinuclear pattern of antineutrophil cytoplasmic antibodies (p-ANCA)	Micropolyarteritis nodosa (PAN) and Churg-Strauss

Name the autoimmune disease of connective tissue associated with the following clinical and pathologic findings:

Keratoconjunctivitis sicca or xerophthalmia, xerostomia, and evidence of other connective tissue disease	Sjögren syndrome
Myositis and heliotrope rash	Dermatomyositis
Rapidly progressive diffuse fibrosis of skin and involved organs including the heart, GI tract, kidney, lung, muscle, and skin	Diffuse scleroderma
CREST syndrome	Localized scleroderma
Disease of connective tissue that lacks renal involvement	Mixed connective tissue disease

What is the most common cause of death due to scleroderma?	Renal crisis (occurs in 50% deaths from scleroderma; treat with ACE inhibitors)
Name the group of disorders characterized by extracellular deposition of protein in a β-pleated sheet conformation:	Amyloidosis (birefringence with Congo Red stain)

Name the effect of amyloidosis on
each of the following organs:

Kidneys	Glomerular, peritubular, and vascular hyalinization
Liver	Hepatomegaly (amyloid deposition in space of Disse)
Heart	Restrictive cardiomyopathy
Tongue	Hypertrophy due to amyloid deposition

Make the Diagnosis

25-y/o male presents with morning stiffness, heel pain, and photophobia; PE: ↓ lumbar spine extension and lateral flexion, tenderness over lumbar spinous processes and iliac crests; w/u: HLA-B27 ⊕; XR: bamboo spine

Ankylosing spondylitis

50-y/o female presents with long-standing h/o morning stiffness and diffuse joint pain; PE: boutonierre and swan neck deformities of fingers, shoulder tenderness and ↓ range of motion (ROM), symmetric and bilateral knee swelling; w/u: RF ⊕

Rheumatoid arthritis (RA)

25-y/o male with a h/o urethritis 2 weeks ago presents with unilateral knee pain, stiffness, and eye pain; PE: conjunctivitis, edema and tenderness of left knee, mucoid urethral discharge; w/u: urethral swab is ⊕ for *Chlamydia.*

Reiter syndrome

45-y/o female presents with dry eyes and dry mouth, PE: parotid gland enlargement; w/u: ⊕ ANA, RF, SS-A/Ro titers

Sjögren syndrome

70-y/o female presents with pain in hands that is worse after activity; PE: Heberden's nodes and Bouchard's nodes, bony enlargement at DIP joints, right knee effusion; w/u: RF and ESR are WNL; XR: joint space narrowing, osteophytes

Osteoarthritis (OA)

72-y/o female presents with a 6-week h/o morning stiffness in neck and shoulders; PE: low-grade fever, tenderness to palpation plus ↓ ROM in neck, shoulder, and hip joints; w/u: ↑ ESR, CRP, RF negative

Polymyalgia rheumatica

50-y/o male presents with acute onset of sharp pain in the left great toe; PE: severe tenderness, swelling, and warmth of the left MTP joint; synovial fluid analysis shows negatively-birefringent crystals.

Gout

25-y/o black female with a 1-week h/o pain in several joints presents with swelling, redness, and pain in her right knee; PE: pustular lesions on palms, right knee shows erythema, tenderness, and ↓ ROM; w/u: gram-negative diplococci in synovial fluid

Gonococcal arthritis

28-y/o female presents with difficulty keeping her eyelids open and holding her head up during the day; PE: weakness of facial muscles, deltoids; ⊕ anti-ACh titer; CXR: anterior mediastinal mass

Myasthenia gravis (associated with thymoma)

25-y/o female with h/o Raynaud's phenomenon presents with arthralgias and myositis; w/u: esophageal hypomotility and ↑ anti-nRNP titers

Mixed connective tissue disease

20-y/o black female presents with fatigue, arthralgias, Raynaud's phenomenon, and pleuritic chest pain; PE: butterfly malar facial rash; w/u: ↓ platelets, proteinuria, and ⊕ ANA, anti-dsDNA, and anti-Smith Abs

SLE

20-y/o with a h/o developmental delay presents with facial weakness; PE: cataracts, marked weakness in muscles of hand, neck, and distal leg, with sustained muscle contraction; genetic testing: cytosine-thymine-guanine (CTG) repeat expansion within DMPK gene

Myotonic dystrophy

DERMATOLOGY

Basic Vocabulary

Give the dermatologic term for each of the following descriptions:

Flat, nonpalpable lesion <1 cm in diameter; different colors that surround skin	Macule
A macule >1 cm in diameter	Patch
Palpable, elevated skin lesion <1 cm in diameter	Papule
A papule >1 cm in diameter	Plaque
Minute, pinpoint, nonblanching hemorrhagic spots in the skin	Petechiae

Similar to petechiae, but larger	Purpura
Fluid-containing blister <0.5 cm in diameter	Vesicle
Fluid-containing blister >0.5 cm in diameter	Bulla
Blister containing pus	Pustule
Solid, round lesion; diameter = thickness	Nodule
Leathery induration of skin caused by scratching	Lichenification
Thickening of the stratum corneum	Hyperkeratosis

Infections

For each of the following descriptions, name the lesion and the treatment of choice:

Inflammation of pilosebaceous unit by *Propionibacterium*, causing comedones and pustules; ↑ during puberty and adolescence	Acne vulgaris **Tx:** topical antibiotics, Retin-A, benzoyl peroxide, isotretinoin if scarring
Honey-colored, crusty vesicles commonly occurring around the mouth and nose in children; caused by *Staphylococcus aureus* or *Streptococcus pyogenes*	Impetigo **Tx:** wash with warm cloth; Keflex or oxacillin for 7-10 days
Subcutaneous, soft-tissue infection with classic signs of inflammation; caused by *Staphylococcus aureus* or *Streptococcus pyogenes*	Cellulitis **Tx:** Keflex or dicloxacillin for 7-10 days
Erythematous rash along major skin folds; more common in diabetics; caused by *Corynebacterium*	Erythrasma **Tx: erythro**mycin
Umbilicated, pearly, dome-shaped papules typically occurring in the genitals; viral etiology	Molluscum contagiosum **Tx:** cryotherapy or trichloroacetic acid (many resolve spontaneously without treatment)
Tender red nodules on the anterior tibial area bilaterally 2° to panniculitis; due to infections, drugs, or inflammatory bowel disease	Erythema nodosum **Tx:** NSAIDs; treat underlying cause

"Sunburn with goosebumps" appearance, Pastia line, strawberry tongue; caused by *S. pyogenes*

Scarlet fever

Tx: penicillin

Small pink papules in groups of 10–20 on the trunk; found in 30% of patients with *Salmonella typhi*

Rose spots

Tx: cholecystectomy for chronic carrier state

Suppurative inflammation of the nail fold surrounding the nail plate; may be due to staphylococcal and streptococcal infection

Paronychia

Tx: warm compress; Keflex if severe

Infection along a fascial plane causing severe pain and inflammation; caused by *S. pyogenes* or *C. perfringens*

Necrotizing fasciitis

Tx: extensive surgical debridement plus clindamycin and penicillin

Obstructed apocrine sweat glands that become infected

Hidradenitis suppurativa

Tx: surgical debridement and antibiotics

Recurrent, vesicular eruptions that occur in groups and are painful; commonly found at oral-labial or genital locations; diagnose with Tzanck smear

Herpes simplex

Tx: oral acyclovir (IV if immunocompromised)

Benign papilloma of viral etiology, most commonly on dorsum of hand; characteristic koilocytes

Verruca vulgaris (common wart)

Tx: cryotherapy or salicylic acid

Contagious, pruritic, "dewdrop" vesicles that occur in kids and can be reactivated into a painful, dermatomal distribution in adults

Varicella (chickenpox and shingles)

Tx: acyclovir for shingles; self-limited in healthy kids; varicella vaccine available for immunocompromised

Pruritic papules in pubic area, buttocks, and axilla caused by lice

Crabs (Pediculosis pubis)

Tx: permethrin 5% shampoo

Contagious, erythematous, pruritic papules, and burrows in intertriginous areas caused by mites

Scabies (Sarcoptes scabiei)

Tx: permethrin 5% cream for patient and close contacts; wash bedding with hot water

Ring-shaped, pruritic, erythematous plaque with elevated borders; caused by fungus

Tinea (corporis if on body; capitis if on head)

Tx: topical antifungal; oral for tinea capitis or resistant lesions

Erythematous scaling patches with satellite pustules, found in intertriginous areas of adults and diaper areas in infants	*Candida* **Tx:** reduce moisture; topical nystatin
Sharply demarcated, *hypopigmented* macules with characteristic "spaghetti and meatball" appearance on KOH prep	Tinea versicolor **Tx:** selenium sulfide shampoo or topical antifungal

Pigmentary Lesions

Name the dermatologic disease or finding associated with each of the following descriptions:

AR defect in melanin synthesis (though melanocytes are present); predisposition to multiple skin disorders	Albinism (oculocutaneous)
Acquired loss of melanocytes → depigmented white patches	Vitiligo
Mask-like facial hyperpigmentation associated with pregnancy	Melasma (chloasma)
Pigmented macules caused by melanocyte hyperplasia; do not darken with sunlight (unlike freckles)	Lentigo
Benign, localized overgrowth of melanin-forming cells of the skin present at birth	Nevocellular nevus
Atypical, irregularly pigmented lesion may evolve into malignant melanoma	Dysplastic nevus
Common benign neoplasm of older adults; sharply demarcated plaques with a pasted on appearance	Seborrheic keratosis (senile keratosis)
Yellowish papules or nodules that tend to occur on the eyelids; associated with hypercholesterolemia	Xanthoma (on the eyelids: xanthelasma)
Hyperpigmentation in the flexural areas that may suggest visceral malignancy	Acanthosis nigricans

Abnormal proliferation of connective tissue that may follow skin trauma; results in large, raised tumor-like scar	Keloid
Capillary hemangioma appearing as a purple-red area on the face or neck	Port-wine stain
Autoimmune disorder presenting with heliotropic patches on eyelids	Dermatomyositis
Erythematous rash that can appear in Christmas tree distribution and is preceded by a herald patch	Pityriasis rosea
Hyperpigmentation, cirrhosis, diabetes mellitus, OA of MCP joints	Hemochromatosis

Name the neurocutaneous syndrome characterized by each of the following features:

Port-wine stains of the face, ipsilateral glaucoma, retinal lesions, and hemangiomas of the meninges	Sturge-Weber syndrome
Hypopigmented macules (ash-leaf spots), adenoma sebaceum, seizures, and mental retardation	Tuberous sclerosis
Multiple organ hemangioblastomas, cysts, and paragangliomas	von Hippel-Lindau disease
Café-au-lait spots, acoustic neuromas, and meningiomas	Neurofibromatosis

Miscellaneous Dermatologic Diseases

Name the blistering dermal disease associated with each of the following descriptions:

Tense, hard subepidermal bullae that tend to occur in the elderly; antiepidermal BM Abs	Bullous pemphigoid
Pruritic subepidermal blisters occurring in groups; eosinophils and IgA deposits at tips of dermal papillae; seen in celiac disease	Dermatitis herpetiformis

Large intraepidermal blisters that often rupture and slough off (Nikolsky's sign); can be fatal; antibodies to desmoglein	Pemphigus vulgaris
Hypersensitivity reaction causing characteristic diffuse, multishaped "target" lesions	Erythema multiforme
Severe-febrile form of erythema multiforme characterized by systemic toxicity, hemorrhagic crusting, and oral mucosal involvement	Stevens-Johnson syndrome
AD defect in heme synthesis; blisters on sun-exposed areas of skin; urine fluoresces orange-pink color with Wood's lamp examination	Porphyria cutanea tarda
What inflammatory disorder is characterized by silvery scaling plaques over the knees, elbows, and scalp?	Psoriasis
Name three classic clinical findings in psoriasis:	1. Fingernail pitting 2. Auspitz sign (removal of scale causes pinpoint bleeding) 3. Koebner phenomenon (lesions appear at sites of cutaneous trauma)
What is the treatment of choice for psoriasis?	First line: topical steroids; second line: PUVA (Psoralens plus UVA light rays)

For each of the following descriptions, name the lesion and the treatment of choice:

Pruritic, inflammatory disorders due to an inherited state of hypersensitivity to environmental allergens	Atopic dermatitis **Tx:** steroids/antihistamines for symptomatic relief
Linear, pruritic rash caused by type IV hypersensitivity reaction to previously sensitized substance	Contact dermatitis **Tx:** topical steroids; antihistamines and systemic steroids for severe cases
Greasy, erythematous scaling patches of the scalp, face, and ears; "cradle cap" in infants	Seborrheic dermatitis **Tx:** selenium sulfide or zinc pyrithione shampoo for scalp, face, and trunk; steroids if severe

| Intensely pruritic, transient, erythematous, papular wheals caused by mast cell degranulation and histamine release | Urticaria (hives)
Tx: steroids/antihistamines for symptomatic relief |

Skin Cancer

Name the skin malignancy associated with each of the following statements:

Most common skin malignancy	Basal cell carcinoma
Associated with excessive sunlight exposure; arises from dysplastic nevus cells	Malignant melanoma
Associated with arsenic and radiation exposure	Squamous cell carcinoma
Actinic keratosis as a precursor.	Squamous cell carcinoma
Pearly papule with translucent border and fine telangiectasias	Basal cell carcinoma
Small, exophytic nodule with crusting or scaling	Squamous cell carcinoma
S-100 used as a tumor marker	Malignant melanoma
Histopathology characterized by "keratin pearls"	Squamous cell carcinoma
Characterized by radial and vertical growth phases	Malignant melanoma
Characterized by locally aggressive, ulcerating, and hemorrhagic lesions; almost never metastatic	Basal cell carcinoma
Occurs in sun-exposed areas and tends to involve the lower part of the face	Squamous cell carcinoma
Occurs in sun-exposed areas and tends to involve the upper part of the face	Basal cell carcinoma

| What is management for actinic keratosis: | Biopsy; treatment with topical 5-fluorouracil (5-FU) or cryotherapy; prevention with sunscreens |

| Name the ABCDE characteristics of melanomas: | **A**symmetry (benign is symmetric)
Border (benign is smooth)
Color (benign is single color)
Diameter (benign is <6 mm)
Elevation (benign is flat) and **E**nlargement (benign is not growing) |

What is the most important prognostic factor in malignant melanoma?	Depth of invasion
What clinical variant of malignant melanoma has the poorest prognosis?	Nodular melanoma
What clinical variant of malignant melanoma often appears on the hands and feet of dark-skinned people?	Acral-lentiginous melanoma
What chronic progressive lymphoma arises in the skin and initially simulates eczema?	Mycosis fungoides
What syndrome is characterized by mycosis fungoides, erythroderma, and scaling?	Sézary syndrome
What connective tissue cancer presents with reddish-purple macules, plaques, or nodules on the skin and mucosa and is caused by HHV-8?	Kaposi's sarcoma

Name the classic dermatologic finding(s) associated with each of the following diseases:

Gastric adenocarcinoma	Acanthosis nigricans
Addison disease	Hyperpigmentation and striae
Rheumatic fever	Erythema marginatum
Kawasaki syndrome	Erythematous palms and soles; dry, red lips; desquamation of fingertips
Severe chronic renal failure	Uremic frost
Bacterial endocarditis	Osler's nodes (tender, raised lesions on pads of fingers or toes) and Janeway lesions (small, erythematous lesions on palms or soles)
Xeroderma pigmentosum	Dry skin and melanoma
Hypothyroidism	Cool, dry skin with coarse brittle hair
Graves disease	Warm, moist skin with fine hair; pretibial myxedema
von Recklinghausen disease (NFT1)	Multiple café-au-lait spots
Familial hypercholesterolemia	Xanthomas
SLE	Malar rash and photosensitivity
Pellagra	Dermatitis

Name the classic dermatologic finding(s) associated with each of the following infectious diseases:

Anthrax	Vesicular papules covered by black eschar
Parvovirus B_{19}	Erythema infectiosum (*slapped-cheek* appearance)
Lyme disease	Erythema chronicum migrans
Primary syphilis	Painless chancre
Secondary syphilis	Rash over palms and soles, condyloma latum
Rocky Mountain spotted fever (RMSF)	Rash over palms and soles (migrates centrally)
Congenital CMV	Pinpoint petechial "blueberry muffin" rash
HPV (in genital region)	Condylomata acuminata
Leprosy	Hypopigmented, anesthetic skin patches

Make the Diagnosis

30-y/o male with h/o recurrent sinusitis presents for sterility evaluation; PE: heart sounds are best heard over right side of chest.

Kartagener syndrome

9-y/o with h/o easy bruising and hyperextensible joints presents to the ER after dislocating his shoulder for the fifth time this year.

Ehlers-Danlos syndrome

5-y/o presents to the ER with his sixth bone fracture in the past 2 years; PE: bluish sclera and mild kyphosis; XR: fractures with evidence of osteopenia

Osteogenesis imperfecta (OI)

8-y/o with h/o severe sunburns and photophobia presents to the dermatologist for evaluation of several lesions on the face that have recently changed color and size.

Xeroderma pigmentosum

6-y/o boy presents to the ophthalmology clinic with sudden ↓ visual acuity; PE: unusual body habitus, long and slender fingers, pectus excavatum, and superiorly dislocated lens

Marfan syndrome

36-y/o with h/o celiac disease presents with clusters of erythematous vesicular lesions over the extensor surfaces of the extremities

Dermatitis herpetiformis

5-y/o patient presents with honey-colored crusted lesions at the angle of his mouth; Gram stain of pus: gram-positive cocci in chains

Impetigo

29-y/o HIV ⊕ patient presents with multiple painless pearly-white umbilicated nodules on the trunk and anogenital area.

Molluscum contagiosum

68-y/o fair-skinned farmer presents with large, telangiectatic, and ulcerated nodule on the bridge of the nose.

Basal cell carcinoma

11-y/o presents with bilateral wrist pain and a rash; PE: erythematous, reticular skin rash of the face and trunk with a "slapped-cheek appearance"

Erythema infectiosum

43-y/o female presents with difficulty swallowing; PE: bluish discoloration of the hands and shiny, tight skin over her face and fingers

Progressive systemic sclerosis (scleroderma)

5-y/o-Asian boy presents with fever and diffuse rash including the palms and soles; PE: cervical lymphadenopathy, conjunctival injection, and desquamation of his fingertips; echocardiogram reveals dilation of coronary arteries.

Kawasaki syndrome (mucocutaneous lymph node syndrome)

33-y/o patient presents with itchy, purple plaques over her wrists, forearms, and inner thigh; PE: Wickham striae

Lichen planus

10-y/o presents with fevers and pruritic rash spreading from the trunk to the arms; PE: "teardrop"-shaped vesicles of varying stages

Varicella

29-y/o athlete presents with a red, pruritic skin eruption with an advancing peripheral, creeping border on the forearm; w/u: septate hyphae on KOH scraping

Tinea corporis (ringworm)

73-y/o presents with a painful, unilateral, vesicular rash in the distribution of the CN V$_1$; PE: diminished corneal sensation

Herpes zoster ophthalmicus

31-y/o obese female presents with pruritis in her skin folds; PE: white curd-like concretions beneath the abdominal panniculus; w/u shows budding yeast on 10% KOH prep

Cutaneous candidiasis

PREVENTATIVE MEDICINE, ETHICS, AND BIOSTATISTICS

Preventative Medicine

Describe the appropriate screening intervention for each of the following cancers:

Breast cancer	Self breast examination every month, >20 y/o
	Clinician breast examination every 3 years from 20 to 40 y/o and every year >40 y/o
	Mammography every year from 50 to 69 y/o
Colon cancer	Hemoccult every year >50 y/o
	Flexible sigmoidoscopy every 3-5 years >50 y/o, *or* colonoscopy every 10 years
	Note: if ⊕ FH, start screening 10 years before age of family member with CA at diagnosis.
Prostate cancer	DRE and PSA every year >50 y/o
Endometrial cancer	High-risk patients should be offered biopsy starting at 35 y/o
Cervical cancer	First Pap smear by 3 years after sexual activity or 21 y/o; then every year thereafter
	At 30 y/o, after three consecutive normal Paps → every 2-3 years pelvic examination every 1-3 years from 20 to 40 y/o and every year >40 y/o

Name the adult immunization recommendations for each of the following diseases:

Varicella

Adults without h/o chickenpox or high-risk patients (eg, immunocompromised)

Hepatitis B

All young adults and high-risk patients (including health-care workers)

Pneumococcal

Administer once to patients >65 y/o or those at high risk

Influenza

Annually for patients >50 y/o or those at high risk

Meningococcal

High-risk patients (eg, college students, military personnel)

Measles, mumps, rubella (MMR)

Everyone born after 1956 who has not yet received vaccination

Tetanus

Primary vaccination necessary for everyone; booster indicated every 10 years

Hepatitis A

Travelers, homosexual males, and h/o chronic liver disease or clotting disorder

Note: vaccination takes 3-4 weeks; give IVIG for short-term prophylaxis or h/o exposure.

What vaccines should be avoided in HIV ⊕ and pregnant patients?

Live vaccinations (MMR, oral polio vaccine [OPV], VZV)

Note: MMR should be given if CD4 >500.

What is the regimen of choice for smoking cessation?

Bupropion plus nicotine replacement (12 months abstinence rate >30%; 2 × more than nicotine replacement alone)

Aging, Death, and Dying

Name the changes found in the elderly in each of the following categories:

Psychiatric

Depression and anxiety more common; suicide rate increases.

Sexual

Men: slower erection/ejaculation, ↑ refractory period

Women: vaginal shortening, thinning, and dryness

Note: sexual interest does *not* decrease.

Sleep patterns	↓ REM, slow-wave sleep; ↑ sleep latency, awakenings
Cognitive	↓ learning speed; intelligence stays the same
Name three conditions that would qualify normal bereavement as pathologic grief:	1. Prolonged grief (>1 year) 2. Excessively intense grief (sleep disturbances, significant weight loss, suicidal ideations) 3. Grief that is delayed, inhibited, or denied
Name the Kübler-Ross stages of dying:	1. Denial 2. Anger 3. Bargaining 4. Depression 5. Acceptance **Note:** one or more stages can occur at once and not necessarily in this order.
What term describes a centralized program of palliative and supportive services to dying persons and their families, in the form of physical, psychologic, social, and spiritual care?	Hospice
What is the criterion to qualify for this type of care?	Medically anticipated death within 6 months

Medical Ethics

Name the term used to describe each of the following ethical responsibilities:	
Requires physicians to "do no harm"	Nonmaleficence
Requires physicians to act in the best interests of the patient	Beneficence (may conflict with patient autonomy)
Demands respect for patient privacy and autonomy	Confidentiality
Name two situations in which a physician must compromise patient confidentiality:	1. Potential harm to self (suicide) or to a third party (Tarasoff decision) 2. Legally defined situations (eg, reportable diseases, gunshot wounds, impaired drivers)
What elements are required in order to prove a malpractice claim?	The "**four Ds**": must prove that the physician showed **d**ereliction (deviation from standard of care) of a **d**uty that caused **d**amages **d**irectly to the patient

What are the four key components to informed consent?

The patient must:
1. Understand the health implications of their diagnosis
2. Be informed of risks, benefits, and alternatives to treatment
3. Be aware of outcome if they do not consent
4. Have the right to withdraw consent at any time

Name four exceptions to informed consent:

1. Patient not legally competent to make decisions.
2. In an emergency (implied consent).
3. Patient waives the right to informed consent.
4. Therapeutic privilege-withholding information that would severely harm the patient or undermine decision-making capacity if revealed.

What are five situations in which parent/legal guardian consent is not required to treat a minor?

1. Emergencies
2. STDs
3. Prescription of contraceptives
4. Treatment of EtOH/drug treatment
5. Care during pregnancy

What four criteria qualify a minor as emancipated?

1. If minor is self-supporting
2. If minor is in the military
3. If minor is married
4. If minor is a parent supporting children

What type of directive is based on the incapacitated patient's prior statements and decisions?

Oral advance directive (substituted judgment standard)

What written advance directive gives instructions for the patient's future health care should he/she become incompetent to make decisions?

Living will; specific examples include DNR (do not resuscitate) or DNI (do not intubate)

What document allows the patient to designate a surrogate to make medical decisions in case the patient loses decision-making capacity?

Durable power of attorney (more flexible than a living will)

When are physicians permitted to refuse a family's request for further intervention on behalf of an ill patient?

On grounds of futility (eg, maximal intervention is failing, no rationale for treatment, and treatment will not achieve the goals of care)

Biostatistics and Clinical Trials

For each description, name the proper term and the equation used to calculate the value:

Probability that a person without the disease will be correctly identified

Specificity = TN/(TN + FP)

Probability that a person who tests positive actually has the disease

Positive predictive value = TP/(TP + FP)

Probability that a person who has a disease will be correctly identified

Sensitivity = TP/(TP + FN)

Total number of cases in a population at any given time

Prevalence = (TP + FN)/(entire population)

Number of new cases that arise in a population over a given time interval

Incidence = Prevalence × duration of disease (approximately)

Used in case-control studies to approximate the relative risk if the disease prevalence is too high

Odds ratio = TP × TN/FP × FN

Used in cohort studies to compare incidence rate in exposed group to that in unexposed group

Relative risk = [TP/(TP + FP)]/[FN/(FN + TN)]

Probability that patient with a negative test actually has no disease

Negative predictive value = TN/ (FN + TN)

How are incidence and prevalence related?

Incidence × disease duration → prevalence

Prevalence >incidence for chronic diseases; prevalence = incidence for acute diseases

What quality is desirable for a screening tool?

High sensitivity (**SNOUT:** **S**e**N**sitivity rules **OUT**)

What quality is desirable for a confirmatory test?

High specificity (**SPIN:** **SP**ecificity rules **IN**)

What is the term for a situation where one outcome is more likely to occur than another?

Bias

Name four ways to reduce bias:

1. Placebo
2. Blinded studies (single, double)
3. Crossover studies (each subject is own control)
4. Randomization

Name the type of study associated with the following descriptions:

Observational study where the sample is chosen based on presence/absence of risk factors	Cohort study (eg, → provides relative risk)
Survey of a population at a single point in time; allows for estimate of disease prevalence	Cross-sectional survey
Experimental study comparing benefits of two or more alternative treatments	Clinical trial
Observational study where the sample is chosen based on disease presence/absence	Case-control study (usually retrospective) → provides odds ratio
Assembling data from multiple studies to achieve great statistical power	Meta-analysis

Name the term for each of the following descriptions:

Refers to the reproducibility of a test	Reliability
Refers to the appropriateness of a test (whether the test measures what it is supposed to)	Validity
Absence of random variation in a test; consistency and reproducibility of a test	Precision
Closeness of a measurement to the truth	Accuracy
Hypothesis postulating that there is no difference between groups	Null hypothesis (H_0)
Error of mistakenly rejecting H_0 (stating that there is a difference when there really is not)	Type I error (α)
Error of failing to reject H_0 (stating there is no difference when there really is)	Type II error (β)
Probability of rejecting H_0 when it is in fact false	Power ($1-\beta$)
Probability of making an α error	P value
Test that compares the difference between two means	t test

Test that analyzes the variance of three or more variables	Analysis of variance (ANOVA)
Test that compares percentages or proportions	χ^2
Absolute value that indicates the strength of a relationship	r (always between –1 and 1)

Name the type of bias described in each of the following examples:

Responses to subjective questions are influenced by knowing what leg of the study a patient is enrolled	Observational bias
Confounding variables introduced by errors of memory made by participants asked to remember past events	Recall bias
Occurs when subjects are assigned to a study group in a nonrandom fashion	Enrollment bias
Bias that is dependent on the rate of disease progression; may lead to overestimation of screening effectiveness in disease	Length bias
Occurs when a patient chooses to enroll in a particular study	Self-selection bias
Occurs when screening tends to prolong the time between diagnosis and death without actually affecting true survival	Lead-time bias

Epidemiology

What is the leading cause of mortality in each of the following age groups:

<1 year	Congenital anomalies
1-14 years	Trauma injuries
15-24 years	Trauma (mostly car accidents)
25-64 years	Cancer (#1 lung, #2 breast/prostate, #3 colon)
≥65 years	Cardiovascular disease

CHAPTER 2

Surgery

TRAUMA

Shock

Define shock:	Inadequate tissue perfusion
What are the four main types of shock?	1. Cardiogenic 2. Septic 3. Hypovolemic 4. Neurogenic

Name the type of shock described below and give the appropriate management:

Hypotension, ↑ pulmonary capillary wedge pressure (PCWP), ↓ cardiac output (CO)	Cardiogenic (usually left ventricular failure) **Treatment/therapy (Tx):** inotropic agents, afterload reduction
Tachycardia, ↓ systolic BP, ↓ pulse pressure	Hypovolemic (usually secondary [2°] to hemorrhage or burns) **Tx:** IV fluid replacement with isotonic Ringer lactate (LR) or normal saline (NS); controlling hemorrhage if applicable
Tachycardia, hypotension, ↑ CO, warm skin with full pulses, fever	Septic (usually 2° to gram-negative organisms) **Tx:** Aggressive IV fluids, antibiotics, vasopressors as needed
Hypotension and bradycardia	Neurogenic (loss of sympathetic tone) **Tx:** IV fluids, vasopressors and identification of neurologic deficits

What are the first five steps in the assessment of a trauma patient?

1. **Airway**: secure airway while maintaining cervical spine stability.
2. **Breathing**: inspect for air movement; assess oxygenation and ventilation.
3. **Circulation**: assess pulses, HR, BP; secure IV access.
4. **Disability**: diagnose neurologic deficits and estimate Glasgow Coma Scale (GCS).
5. **Exposure/environment**: complete visual inspection and palpation of patient while maintaining normal body temperature.

Name the diagnosis associated with each of the following findings:

Hemotympanum, clear otorrhea/ rhinorrhea, raccoon eyes, and Battle sign

Basilar skull fracture (Fx)

Ecchymosis of lower abdomen from seatbelt (seatbelt sign)

Small bowel perforation (in 20% of cases)

Hypotension, jugular venous distension (JVD), decreased heart sounds

Beck triad (seen in cardiac tamponade and tension pneumothorax)

Beck triad and pulsus paradoxus

Cardiac tamponade

Unilateral absence of breath sounds, JVD, mediastinal shift

Tension pneumothorax

Paradoxical chest wall movement

Flail chest (multiple rib Fx with pulmonary injury)

GENERAL SURGERY

Esophagus

What is the common presentation of *oropharyngeal* dysphagia?

Difficulty swallowing liquids > solids

What is the common presentation of *esophageal* dysphagia?

Difficulty swallowing *both* liquids and solids

What is the common presentation of dysphagia secondary to mechanical obstruction?

Difficulty swallowing solids > liquids

What is the differential diagnosis of oropharyngeal dysphagia?

Zenker diverticulum, neurologic disorders (cranial nerves, muscles), sphincter dysfunction, and neoplasm

What term is used to describe a false diverticulum above the cricopharyngeus muscle?	Zenker diverticulum
What two tests are essential in the evaluation of oropharyngeal dysphagia?	Barium swallow followed by endoscopy if no diverticulum is seen
What is the risk of endoscopy with oropharyngeal dysphagia?	Risk of esophageal perforation is high with Zenker diverticulum. **Note:** Zenker diverticulum must be ruled out with a barium swallow.
What is the treatment of a Zenker diverticulum?	Myotomy ± excision of diverticulum
What is the differential diagnosis for esophageal dysphagia?	1. Achalasia 2. Esophageal stricture 3. Lower esophageal web 4. Scleroderma 5. Esophageal cancer

Name the esophageal disease associated with the following characteristics:

Inability of the lower esophageal sphincter (LES) to relax with loss of esophageal peristalsis; "bird beak" appearance on barium swallow and ↑ resting pressure of LES on manometry	Achalasia (ganglionic loss of Auerbach plexus)
May result from ingestion of caustic agents (eg, lye, oven cleaners, batteries, or drain cleaners)	Esophageal stricture
Syndrome characterized by iron-deficiency anemia, dysphagia, esophageal web, and atrophic glossitis	Plummer-Vinson syndrome
Columnar metaplasia of squamous epithelium of the distal esophagus in response to prolonged injury (often 2° to long-standing gastroesophageal reflux disease [GERD])	Barrett esophagus
What type of malignancy occurs in patients with long-standing Barrett esophagus?	Esophageal cancer (usually adenocarcinoma); 10× ↑ risk → rule out with endoscopy

Name six important risk factors for esophageal carcinoma:	**ABCDEF** 1. Achalasia 2. Barrett esophagus 3. Corrosive esophagitis 4. Diverticuli 5. Esophageal webs, ethanol (EtOH) 6. Familial
What are the two main histologic types of esophageal cancer?	Squamous cell carcinoma and adenocarcinoma near the gastroesophageal (GE) junction
What type of esophageal cancer is associated with alcohol and tobacco use?	Squamous cell carcinoma
Barrett esophagus is a risk factor for what type of esophageal cancer?	Adenocarcinoma
What diagnostic test is necessary in the workup (w/u) for all patients with suspected esophageal cancer?	Esophagogastroduodenoscopy (EGD) with tissue biopsy
What diagnosis must be ruled out in a patient with sudden onset severe retrosternal chest pain that is worse with swallowing and deep inhalation following EGD?	Esophageal perforation
What syndrome is characterized by esophageal perforation following severe vomiting?	Boerhaave syndrome
What is the difference between Boerhaave and Mallory-Weiss tears?	Mallory-Weiss: superficial tears in the esophageal mucosa; Boerhaave: full-thickness esophageal rupture
What term is used to describe the crunching sound heard with each heartbeat in a patient with mediastinal emphysema?	Hamman's sign
What tests are used to make a definitive diagnosis of esophageal perforation?	Chest x-ray (CXR) (showing mediastinal/subcutaneous air, pneumothorax, left pleural effusion) and esophagogram
What is the treatment of esophageal perforation?	Thoracotomy, primary repair, and drainage within 24 h (>50% mortality if treatment delayed)

What disease is characterized by substernal chest pain, heartburn, and regurgitation, commonly worse after meals and in the supine position?	GERD
What pulmonary condition has associated symptoms that may also be seen in patients with GERD?	Asthma (wheezing/cough/dyspnea)
Name the six major risk factors for GERD:	1. Obesity 2. Pregnancy 3. Alcohol 4. Caffeine 5. Smoking (nicotine) 6. Fatty food diet
Name three diseases closely associated with GERD:	1. Sliding hiatal hernia 2. Scleroderma 3. Achalasia
Name three diagnostic studies that can be used to make a diagnosis of GERD:	1. EGD 2. pH probe 3. Barium swallow
What condition is a major concern in patients with long-standing GERD?	Barrett's esophagus (metaplasia of distal esophagus)
What is the medical treatment for Barrett's esophagus?	Antacids, H_2 blockers, or proton pump inhibitors (PPi) with surveillance EGD and biopsies
Name five possible complications of GERD:	1. Ulceration 2. Stricture formation 3. Barrett's esophagus 4. Bleeding 5. Aspiration of gastric contents
What are the indications for surgery in a patient with GERD?	Failure of medical treatment, stricture formation, severe dysphasia, and Barrett's esophagus

Stomach

What disease is characterized by erosion of the gastric or duodenal mucosa?	Peptic ulcer disease (PUD)
What are the classic symptoms associated with PUD?	Epigastric pain relieved with antacids, nausea, "coffee-ground" emesis, melena, and hematochezia

What is the differential diagnosis of epigastric pain?	1. PUD 2. Gastritis 3. Pancreatitis 4. Cholecystitis 5. Coronary artery disease (CAD) 6. GERD
What pathogen is found in >90% of patients with duodenal ulcers and 70% of patients with gastric ulcer disease?	*Helicobacter pylori*
Aside from *H. pylori* infection, name four other common risk factors for PUD:	1. NSAIDs 2. EtOH 3. Smoking 4. Corticosteroids
What study is used to definitively diagnose PUD?	EGD with biopsies (for *H. pylori* and to rule out gastric cancer)
What is the most common location of a *gastric* ulcer?	Body of the stomach
What is the most common location of a *duodenal* ulcer?	First part of the duodenum

Name the type of peptic ulcer (gastric or duodenal) associated with each of the following findings:

Pain is worse during meals	Gastric ulcer (pain is **G**reater with meals) → weight loss
Pain improves after meals	**D**uodenal ulcer (pain **D**ecreases with meals) → weight gain
Almost 100% associated with *H. pylori* infection	Duodenal ulcer
NSAIDs, alcohol use, and smoking are implicated in pathogenesis	Gastric ulcer
Gastric acid production may be reduced	Gastric ulcer
Associated with Zollinger-Ellison syndrome; ↑ serum gastrin levels	Duodenal ulcer
Most common type of PUD	Duodenal ulcer (twice as common as gastric ulcers)
Occur in the setting of ↓ mucosal protection against gastric acid	Both

What are the four treatment goals for PUD?	1. Decrease acid production 2. Mucosal protection 3. Eradication of *H. pylori* 4. Cancer surveillance (gastric)
What medications are used for acid suppression?	H_2 blockers and PPi
What medications are used for mucosal protection?	Sucralfate, bismuth, and misoprostol
What is the treatment for *H. pylori*?	"Triple therapy" (PPi, bismuth salicylate, and two of the following antibiotics: metronidazole, amoxicillin, clarithromycin, or tetracycline); requires 6-8 weeks to heal
What diagnostic study must be performed in patients with nonhealing gastric ulcers?	EGD with biopsy (must rule out gastric adenocarcinoma)
Name three common complications of PUD requiring intervention:	1. Hemorrhage from erosion of an ulcer into a blood vessel 2. Perforation 3. Obstruction
What are the classic symptoms of gastric outlet obstruction?	Nausea/vomiting (N/V), crampy abdominal pain, weight loss, and distended/dilated stomach
What is the typical presentation of a perforated ulcer?	Sudden, severe onset abdominal pain radiating to back and shoulders, N/V, and peritoneal signs (rebound tenderness, guarding, and motion pain on examination)
What finding on x-ray is an absolute indication for surgery?	Free air under the diaphragm
What is the treatment of a perforated duodenal ulcer?	Nothing by mouth (NPO), IV fluids (IVF), antibiotics, and surgery
What is a life-threatening complication of a posterior duodenal ulcer?	Massive hemorrhage from erosion into the gastroduodenal artery
What are the key steps in the initial management of any patient with a severe upper GI bleed?	ABCs, IV fluids (via bilateral large peripheral IVs), nasogastric tube (NGT) suction, gastric lavage, blood transfusion if necessary

What is the most important diagnostic imaging test in a patient with a severe upper GI bleed?	Endoscopy
What type of treatment can be administered during endoscopy in a patient with an upper GI bleed?	Injection of bleeding vessel with sclerosing or vasoconstrictive agents
What type of treatment is indicated in patients with GI bleeding refractory to endoscopic treatment?	Surgery
What is the differential diagnosis of an upper GI bleed?	1. Duodenal ulcer (40%) 2. Gastric ulcer (10%-20%) 3. Gastritis (15%-20%), 4. Varices (10%) 5. Mallory-Weiss tear (10%)
What term is used to describe a small esophageal tear near the GE junction, commonly occurring after retching, that may cause minor self-limited upper GI bleeding?	Mallory-Weiss tear
What cause of upper GI bleeding has the highest potential for rapid, life-threatening exsanguination?	Esophageal varices

Name the type of ulcer defined below:

Acute gastric ulcer found in burn and trauma victims	Curling's ulcer
Acute gastric ulcer associated with head trauma or surgery causing elevated intracranial pressure	Cushing's ulcer
Ulcer at a GI anastomotic site	Marginal ulcer

Name the type of gastritis associated with the following findings:

Autoimmune disorder with Autoantibodies to parietal cells and intrinsic factor (IF), Achlorhydria, pernicious Anemia, and Aging	Type A (fundal) chronic gastritis (remember the five A's for Type A)
"Coffee-ground" emesis from mucosal inflammation	Acute (stress) gastritis
H. pylori infection	Type B (antral) chronic gastritis (B = bug)
NSAID ingestion	Type B (antral) chronic gastritis

Increased risk of PUD and gastric carcinoma	Type B (antral) chronic gastritis
Critically ill patients	Acute (stress) gastritis

What percentage of gastric tumors are malignant?	90%-95% (95% are carcinomas)
What are the most common presenting symptoms in a patient with gastric carcinoma?	Pain, anorexia, and weight loss
What are the major risk factors for gastric carcinoma?	Age >60, diet rich in nitrites and salts and low in fresh vegetables, and chronic gastritis
What histopathologic finding in gastric cancer is associated with prognosis?	Depth of invasion
What is the diagnostic test of choice in a patient with suspected gastric carcinoma?	EGD with biopsies and endoscopic ultrasound to determine depth of invasion and nodal metastases
What are the three main patterns of gastric tumor growth?	1. Ulcerating (most common) 2. Fungating 3. Diffusely infiltrating (linitis plastica)

Provide the term associated with each of the following statements about gastric carcinoma metastases:

Metastases to the pouch of Douglas in the pelvis	Blumer shelf
Metastases to the ovary	Krukenberg tumor
Metastases to the left supraclavicular fossa	Virchow node
Periumbilical lymph node metastases	Sister Mary Joseph node

Gallbladder

What are the risk factors for cholelithiasis?	**Four F's:** Fertile, Fat, Forty years old, and Female
What is the typical presentation of cholelithiasis?	Postprandial right upper quadrant (RUQ) pain (usually after fatty meals) with N/V
What are the two types of stones found in the gallbladder?	1. Cholesterol (75%) 2. Pigment stones (25%)

Name the type of gallstone associated with each of the following:

Native American	Cholesterol stone
Congenital hemoglobinopathy, hemolytic anemia	Pigment stone
Radiopaque	Pigment stone
Crohn's disease, cystic fibrosis	Cholesterol stone
Rapid weight loss (ie, post-gastric bypass)	Cholesterol stone

What is the diagnostic test for cholelithiasis?

RUQ ultrasound (98% sensitive and specific!)

What are five possible complications of cholelithiasis?

1. Acute cholecystitis
2. Choledocholithiasis
3. Gallstone pancreatitis
4. Gallstone ileus
5. Cholangitis

What is the treatment for symptomatic cholelithiasis?

Elective cholecystectomy

What are the indications for surgery in an asymptomatic patient?

Sickle cell disease and porcelain gallbladder ($\uparrow$ risk of CA)

What term is used to describe prolonged blockage of the cystic duct by an impacted stone leading to inflammation, infection, and possible gangrene of the gallbladder?

Acute cholecystitis

How does the pain differ in cholecystitis compared to cholelithiasis?

Pain in cholecystitis is more severe and prolonged.

What physical examination finding is characterized by inspiratory arrest upon deep palpation of the RUQ in cholecystitis?

Murphy's sign (acute cholecystitis)

What are the other common signs and symptoms of cholecystitis?

Fever, N/V, tender gallbladder, leukocytosis, and referred right subscapular pain

What are three common findings on ultrasound (US) in a patient with acute cholecystitis?

1. Gallbladder wall thickening
2. Pericholecystic fluid
3. Presence of stones

What test may be done in a patient with acute cholecystitis when the ultrasound (US) is equivocal?

Hepatobiliary iminodiacetic acid (HIDA) scan (failure to visualize the gallbladder $\rightarrow$ acute cholecystitis)

What is the treatment of acute cholecystitis?	IVF, antibiotics, and early (<72 h) or late (6 weeks) cholecystectomy
Define choledocholithiasis:	Presence of gallstones within the common bile duct
What is the treatment for choledocholithiasis?	1. Endoscopic retrograde cholangiopancreatography (ERCP) with papillotomy and stone removal 2. Common bile duct exploration
What are two common complications of choledocholithiasis?	Cholangitis and pancreatitis
What is cholangitis?	Infection of the biliary tree 2° to obstruction
What are the two most common causes of bile duct obstruction?	1. Gallstones 2. Malignancy
Name five classic signs and symptoms of obstructive jaundice:	1. Jaundice 2. Pruritus 3. Dark urine 4. Clay-colored stool 5. Weight loss (chronic)
What is Charcot's triad of cholangitis?	1. RUQ pain 2. Jaundice 3. Fever/chills
What is Reynold's pentad of cholangitis?	Charcot's triad + shock and altered mental status
What is Courvoisier's sign?	Painless enlargement of the gallbladder with jaundice caused by carcinoma of the head of the pancreas
What are the common lab abnormalities in a patient with cholangitis?	Leukocytosis, ↑ direct bilirubin, and ↑ alkaline phosphatase (sensitive for bile duct inflammation)
What is the diagnostic gold standard for cholangitis?	ERCP
What organism most commonly causes cholangitis?	*Escherichia coli*
What is the treatment for cholangitis?	IVF, antibiotics, and relief of obstruction (ERCP with papillotomy, percutaneous transhepatic cholangiography [PTC] with catheter placement, or surgery)

Name two important complications of chronic cholangitis:	1. Cholangiocarcinoma 2. Cirrhosis
What is the common comorbidity in patients with sclerosing cholangitis?	Inflammatory bowel disease (60%)
What is the surgical treatment of sclerosing cholangitis?	Removal of extrahepatic bile ducts (due to ↑ CA risk) and hepatoenteric anastomosis or transplant procedure
What is the most common type of gallbladder malignancy?	Adenocarcinoma (90%)
What are the major risk factors for gallbladder cancer?	Gallstones and porcelain gallbladder (10% have CA)
What is the name for malignancy of the intra- or extrahepatic bile ducts?	Cholangiocarcinoma
What are the major risk factors for cholangiocarcinoma?	Ulcerative colitis, sclerosing cholangitis, and thorotrast contrast dye
What is the name of a tumor at the junction of the left and right hepatic ducts?	Klatskin tumor
What surgery is typically performed for a distal cholangiocarcinoma?	Whipple procedure (pancreaticoduodenectomy)

Pancreas

Name nine causes of acute pancreatitis:	"GET SMASHeD" 1. **G**allstones 2. **E**thanol, ERCP 3. **T**rauma 4. **S**teroids 5. **M**umps (viruses) 6. **A**utoimmune disorder 7. **S**corpion sting 8. **H**yperlipidemia 9. **D**rugs (especially didanosine [DDI])
What terms are used to refer to periumbilical and flank ecchymoses in hemorrhagic pancreatitis?	Cullen's sign and Grey-Turner sign, respectively

Name six complications of acute pancreatitis:	1. Systemic inflammatory response syndrome (SIRS) 2. Necrosis 3. Pseudocyst formation 4. Pancreatic ascites 5. Fistula formation 6. GI or biliary obstruction
What are two classic radiologic findings on abdominal x-ray (AXR) in acute pancreatitis?	1. A **sentinel loop** of dilated bowel in left upper quadrant (LUQ) next to inflamed pancreas 2. The **colon cutoff sign:** distended transverse colon with an absence of colonic gas distal to the splenic flexure
What is the most appropriate radiologic study for severe pancreatitis?	Abdominal computed tomography (CT)
What other test should be included in the diagnostic w/u of suspected gallstone pancreatitis?	RUQ ultrasound (to look for gallstones)
How many days after a bout of gallstone pancreatitis should a cholecystectomy be performed?	3-5 days after resolution of pancreatitis
In a patient undergoing cholecystectomy for a history of (h/o) gallstone pancreatitis, what test should be done intraoperatively?	Intraoperative cholangiogram (to rule out choledocholithiasis)
How is prognosis estimated in a patient with acute pancreatitis?	Ranson criteria: 0-2 positives (<5% mortality rate), 3-4 (15%), 5-6 (40%), 7-8 (~100%)
What are the Ranson criteria at presentation?	1. Age >55 2. WBC >16,000 3. Glucose >200 mg/dL 4. AST >250 5. LDH >350
What are the Ranson criteria after 48 h?	1. Base deficit >4 2. ↑ in BUN >5 3. Fluid sequestration >6 L 4. Ca^{2+} <8.5 5. ↓ in Hct >10% 6. PaO_2 <60

Name four common laboratory abnormalities in acute pancreatitis:	1. ↑↑ Serum amylase (within 24 h) 2. ↑↑ Serum lipase (72-96 h) 3. Hypocalcemia 4. Glycosuria
What is the difference between a true cyst and a pseudocyst?	A true cyst is lined by epithelial cells, while a pseudocyst is lined by fibrous tissue.
When should a pseudocyst be drained interventionally?	If the cyst is >6 cm for 6 weeks (50% resolve spontaneously), or if it is infected
What are the procedures for interval pseudocyst drainage?	Cystogastrostomy, cystojejunostomy, and cystoduodenostomy
Name five common causes of chronic pancreatitis:	ABCCD 1. **A**lcoholism (#1 in adults) 2. **B**iliary tract disease 3. **C**ystic fibrosis (#1 in kids) 4. **C**a2$^+$ (hypercalcemia) 5. **D**ivisum (pancreas divisum)
What is a classic diagnostic finding seen on AXR in chronic pancreatitis?	Calcification of the pancreas
What are two clinical signs of pancreatic insufficiency?	Diabetes (inadequate endocrine function) and steatorrhea (inadequate exocrine function)
What is the greatest risk factor for pancreatic cancer?	Smoking (3× ↑ risk)
Most pancreatic tumors are found in what region of the pancreas?	Two-thirds of pancreatic tumors are found in the pancreatic head.
What is a common clinical consequence of a mass in the pancreatic head?	Obstructive, painless jaundice causing malabsorption and Courvoisier's (enlarged, palpable) gallbladder
What is Trousseau's *syndrome*?	Migratory superficial thrombophlebitis associated with visceral cancer (commonly pancreatic adenocarcinoma)
What are two serologic markers of pancreatic cancer?	1. Carcinoembryonic antigen (CEA) 2. CA 19-9
What is the prognosis for pancreatic adenocarcinoma?	4% 5-year survival

What surgical procedure is commonly used for resection of a tumor in the head of the pancreas?

Whipple procedure (pancreaticoduodenectomy)

What characteristics of a tumor are contraindications for aggressive surgical intervention?

Vascular encasement, liver metastasis, peritoneal implants, distal lymph node metastasis, and distant metastasis

Liver

Name the most common:

Benign liver tumor

Hemangioma

Primary liver cancer

Hepatocellular carcinoma (hepatoma)

Liver cancer

Metastasis

What is the feared complication of a hepatic hemangioma?

Hemorrhage (*do not* biopsy)

What is the treatment of a hepatic hemangioma?

Observation (surgery only if symptomatic)

What liver tumor is associated with oral contraceptives and anabolic steroids?

Hepatic adenoma

What is the treatment of a hepatic adenoma?

Discontinue birth control pills and observation.

Name the two main types of liver abscesses:

1. Pyogenic
2. Parasitic

What pathogen most frequently causes parasitic abscesses?

Entamoeba histolytica

What are the symptoms of a parasitic abscess caused by *E. histolytica*?

RUQ pain, fever, and bloody diarrhea

What is the treatment of a parasitic abscess?

IV metronidazole (surgery only if refractory)

What diagnosis is suggested by the presence of multiple small hepatic cysts on CT scan?

Infection with *Echinococcus granulosus* (eosinophilia and a ⊕ heme agglutination test are also common)

What procedure is contraindicated in treatment of hydatid disease (*Echinococcal* cysts)?

Aspiration (requires open procedure to avoid contamination of peritoneal) cavity

Name the three most common organisms found in a pyogenic liver abscess:	1. *E. coli* 2. *Klebsiella* 3. *Proteus*
Name the major risk factors for hepatocellular carcinoma:	**"WATCH for ABC"** **W**ilson's disease α-1-**A**ntiTrypsin **C**arcinogens (eg, aflatoxin B_1, polyvinyl chloride) **H**emochromatosis **A**lcoholic cirrhosis Hepatitis **B** Hepatitis **C**
Where is the most common site of metastasis for hepatocellular carcinoma?	Lung
What are the treatment options for hepatocellular carcinoma?	Surgical resection, chemoembolization, local ablation, or transplantation (monitor with α-fetoprotein)

Spleen

What are the indications for splenectomy in a patient with idiopathic thrombocytopenic purpura (ITP)?	Failed corticosteroid treatment
Name three absolute indications for splenectomy:	1. Hereditary spherocytosis 2. Splenic tumors 3. **Massive** splenic trauma or spontaneous rupture
What is the main postsplenectomy complication?	Overwhelming postsplenectomy sepsis (OPSS)
What are the three main organisms responsible for OPSS?	1. *Streptococcus pneumoniae* 2. *Neisseria meningitidis* 3. *Haemophilus influenzae* **Note:** all are **encapsulated.**
What are commonly administered to prevent OPSS?	Vaccinations

Hernias

Name the two factors that contribute to hernia formation:	1. Increased abdominal pressure (heavy lifting, cough, straining, pregnancy, ascites, obesity) 2. Congenital defects

Name the hernia descriptor defined below:

Hernia sac that returns, either spontaneously or after manipulation, to its normal anatomic location	Reducible
Hernia sac that cannot be reduced	Incarcerated
Incarcerated hernia sac causing hernia contents to become ischemic and eventually necrotic	Strangulated (requires emergent surgery)

Name the type of hernia described below:

Inguinal hernia that protrudes from the peritoneal cavity *lateral* to the epigastric vessels; results from a patent processus vaginalis	Indirect inguinal hernia
Inguinal hernia that protrudes from the peritoneal cavity *medial* to the epigastric vessels	Direct inguinal hernia (hernia usually passes through Hasselbach's Hasselbach's triangle 2° to weakness of transversalis fascia)
Hernia protruding through the femoral sheath in the femoral canal medial to the femoral vein	Femoral hernia
Hernia protruding through the esophageal hiatus	Hiatal hernia (commonly leads to acid reflux disease)
Incarcerated hernia involving only one side of the bowel wall	Richter's hernia
Most common hernia in both males and females	Indirect inguinal hernia
Hernia that is more common in females than males	Femoral hernia
Type of hernia that may result in gangrenous bowel without causing small bowel obstruction (SBO)	Richter's hernia

Name three common complications of a hernia:	1. Pain 2. SBO 3. Necrosis of strangulated bowel
What is the definitive treatment for a hernia?	Surgical repair

Small Intestine

What condition commonly presents with abdominal discomfort, N/V, distension, cramping, and high-pitched bowel sounds?	SBO
What are the two most common causes of SBO?	1. Adhesions 2. Hernias
What are five less common causes of SBO?	1. Neoplasms 2. Intussusception 3. Volvulus 4. Gallstone ileus 5. Crohn's disease
What type of hernia needs to be ruled out on physical examination in a patient with suspected SBO?	Incarcerated hernia
What are three common findings in a patient with strangulated bowel?	1. Leukocytosis 2. Tachycardia 3. Peritoneal signs
What is the key component of the history in a patient with suspected SBO?	Previous abdominal surgery (leading to adhesions)
What is the initial management of an adhesive SBO?	NPO, IVF, and NGT suction
What radiographic studies are commonly performed in patients with suspected SBO?	Acute abdominal series (upright AP CXR, upright AXR, and flat-plate AXR)
What are three common findings on AXR in a patient with SBO?	1. Distended loops of bowel 2. Air-fluid levels 3. Paucity of gas in colon/rectum
Define partial SBO:	Incomplete bowel obstruction with the presence of colonic gas
What is the classic acid-base disturbance in SBO?	Hypovolemic hypochloremic hypokalemic alkalosis (secondary to vomiting or nasogastric suction)
Why do patients with SBO develop hypokalemia?	Alkalosis drives K^+ into cells.

What finding on urinalysis is characteristic of SBO?	Paradoxical aciduria
Why does aciduria occur?	H^+ exchanged for Na^+ during fluid resuscitation
What is the treatment of a *partial* SBO?	Conservative management and close monitoring
What is the treatment for a *complete* SBO?	Surgery
What type of obstruction is commonly associated with cramping abdominal pain, distention, nausea, and *feculent* vomitus?	Large bowel obstruction (LBO)
What are the three most common causes of LBO?	1. Colon CA 2. Diverticulitis 3. Volvulus
What is the assumed cause of LBO until proven otherwise?	Colon cancer
What are the three studies necessary in the evaluation of LBO?	1. Contrast enema 2. CT scan 3. Colonoscopy if patient stable

Colon

What are the two most common causes of lower GI bleed (LGIB)?	1. Diverticulosis 2. Angiodysplasia (arteriovenous malformation)
Of the two most common etiologies for LGIB, which is most likely to present with intermittent bleeding?	Angiodysplasia
What is the source of bleeding in diverticular disease?	Erosion of a diverticulum into a colonic blood vessel
In what age group is diverticular disease most common?	>60 years old
What is the most common presenting symptom of diverticulitis?	Left lower quadrant (LLQ) pain
What is the strongest risk factor for diverticular disease?	Low-fiber diet

What is the best radiologic test for the diagnosis of acute diverticulitis?	Abdominal/pelvic CT
What is the most common site of diverticular disease?	Sigmoid colon (95%)
Name four common complications of diverticulitis:	1. Abscess 2. Peritonitis 3. Fistula formation 4. Obstruction
Patients who are status post (s/p) hysterectomy are at increased risk of developing what complication of diverticulitis?	Enterovaginal fistula
What is the treatment of an initial attack of diverticulitis?	NPO, IVF, and antibiotics (ABx) (enteric and anaerobic coverage)
What is the risk of recurrence of an attack of diverticulitis after an initial episode?	33%
When is elective surgery indicated for diverticulitis?	After the second attack or after the first attack in a young, diabetic, or immunosuppressed patient
What must be ruled out in *every* patient with diverticulitis?	Colorectal cancer
What is volvulus and where does it most commonly occur?	Complete twisting of the bowel around its mesenteric base occurring most commonly in the sigmoid colon in elderly patients
How is volvulus diagnosed?	Sigmoidoscopy (also therapeutic for a nonstrangulated volvulus) or contrast enema
What inflammatory disease is often caused by overgrowth of exotoxin-producing bacteria?	Pseudomembranous colitis
What organism is most commonly responsible for pseudomembranous colitis?	*Clostridium difficile*
What tests are used for the diagnosis of pseudomembranous colitis?	Colonoscopy revealing pseudomembranes or *C. difficile* toxin detected in stool

What is the *early* finding in acute mesenteric ischemia? | Abdominal pain out of proportion to examination

What are the *late* findings in acute mesenteric ischemia? | Bloody diarrhea, fever, and peritonitis (80% mortality)

List the three main causes of mesenteric ischemia:
1. Embolization (atrial fibrillation)
2. Thrombosis (atherosclerotic plaque)
3. Nonocclusive ischemia ($\downarrow$ CO or medications)

What is the drug classically associated with mesenteric ischemia? | Digoxin

What is the triad of symptoms in chronic mesenteric ischemia?
1. Postprandial abdominal pain
2. Weight loss
3. Food aversion/fear

How many vessels must be occluded to produce symptomatic chronic mesenteric ischemia? | Two out of three mesenteric arteries (celiac, superior mesenteric artery [SMA], inferior mesenteric artery [IMA])

Ischemic bowel disease commonly affects which part of the GI tract? | "Watershed" areas (splenic flexure, rectosigmoid junction)

What is the diagnostic test of choice for mesenteric ischemia? | Arteriogram

Name the autosomal dominant syndrome associated with each of the following findings:

Colonic polyps, osteomas, and soft tissue tumors; associated with abnormal dentition | Gardner's syndrome

Hundreds of colonic polyps; malignant potential ~100% | Familial adenomatous polyposis (FAP)

Colonic polyps and central nervous system (CNS) tumors; malignant potential ~100% | Turcot's syndrome

Defect in DNA repair → many colonic lesions (especially proximal); malignant potential ~50% | Hereditary nonpolyposis colorectal carcinoma (HNPCC) or Lynch syndrome

Benign hamartomas of GI tract, melanotic pigmentation of hand, mouth, and genitalia; no malignant potential (but ↑ risk of other tumors) | Peutz-Jeghers syndrome

Name the type of neoplastic polyp:

Usually benign and pedunculated; most common type	Tubular adenoma (75%)
Highly malignant, sessile tumor with fingerlike projections	Villous adenoma
Shares features of both other types of polyps	Tubulovillous adenoma

Name five major risk factors for colon cancer:

1. Colonic villous adenomas
2. Inflammatory bowel disease (IBD)
3. ↓ Fiber, ↑ animal fat diet
4. Age >50
5. Positive family/personal history

How does colorectal carcinoma typically present?

Left side lesion → constipation; right side lesion → anemia (from occult blood loss)

In an older adult male with iron-deficiency anemia what diagnosis must be ruled out?

Colon cancer (second most common cancer in the United States)

What is the current recommendation for colon cancer screening?

Hemoccult and digital rectal examination (DRE) every year >50 y/o

Flexible sigmoidoscopy every 3-5 years >50 y/o, *or* colonoscopy every 10 years

Note: if ⊕ family history (FH), start screening 10 years before the age of the family member with CA at diagnosis.

What is the gold standard for the diagnosis of colon cancer?

Colonoscopy with tissue biopsy

How does rectal CA usually present?

Hematochezia, tenesmus, and incomplete evacuation of stool

What is the primary therapy for colorectal cancer?

Surgical resection (adjuvant therapy for Stage III)

What marker can be used to follow progression of colon cancer treatment?

CEA

Note: CEA is not specific enough to serve as an adequate screening method.

Appendix

What are the two most common causes of appendiceal obstruction?	Obstruction of the appendix due to fecalith and lymphoid hyperplasia
What is the classic presentation of appendicitis?	Acute onset of periumbilical pain (referred pain) followed by N/V, *anorexia,* and right lower quadrant (RLQ) pain (due to localized peritoneal irritation)
In what order do patients with appendicitis typically experience the symptoms of abdominal pain and N/V?	Pain precedes N/V in appendicitis. **Note:** nausea and vomiting followed by abdominal pain suggests gastroenteritis.
How is the diagnosis of appendicitis made?	By history and physical examination
What are the classic physical examination findings in a patient with appendicitis?	Low-grade fever, RLQ pain with local signs of peritoneal irritation (guarding, rebound tenderness)
What lab tests are typically ordered in the w/u of appendicitis?	CBC (leukocytosis), urinalysis (r/o UTI or calculus), and β-hCG (all female patients)
What radiologic test can be done when the diagnosis of appendicitis is in doubt?	Abdominal/pelvic CT **Note:** ultrasound is recommended in children and pregnant woman.
What is the best radiologic test for evaluation of ovarian causes of lower abdominal pain?	Ultrasound
What is the most common emergency abdominal surgery performed in the United States?	Appendectomy
Name each physical examination finding described below:	
Point of maximal tenderness one-third the distance from the anterior iliac spine to the umbilicus	McBurney's point
Pain in RLQ on palpation of LLQ	Rovsing's sign
Pain on internal rotation of the leg with both hip and knee flexed	Obturator sign
Pain on extension of hip with knee in full flexion	Psoas sign

What is the treatment of appendicitis?	IVF, antibiotics, and surgery
What are two common feared complications of ruptured appendicitis?	1. Peritonitis 2. Abscess formation
How is an abscess caused by appendicitis managed?	Percutaneous drainage, antibiotics, and interval appendectomy 6-8 weeks later
How long should a patient with appendicitis be treated with antibiotics?	24 h (nonperforated), 7-10 days (perforated)
What is the most common tumor of the appendix?	Carcinoid tumor
What type of cells give rise to carcinoid tumors?	Neuroendocrine (Kulchitsky) cells
What substances are secreted from carcinoid tumors?	Serotonin, histamine, and prostaglandins
What type of carcinoid tumors tend to be the most aggressive?	Ileal, gastric, and colonic
Name five clinical findings of carcinoid syndrome:	1. Vasomotor dysfunction 2. GI hypermotility 3. Bronchoconstriction 4. Hepatomegaly 5. Right-sided heart valve degeneration
Metastasis of a carcinoid tumor to what organ may result in carcinoid syndrome?	Liver
What lab test is used to diagnose carcinoid syndrome?	5-hydroxyindoleacetic acid (5-HIAA) in urine
What is the treatment for a carcinoid tumor?	Surgical resection (octreotide for carcinoid syndrome)

Breast

What is the second leading cause of cancer death among women?	Breast cancer
Name five risk factors for breast cancer:	1. Older age 2. FH of premenopausal breast cancer 3. Nulliparity 4. Age of menarche <13 or age at menopause <55 5. First pregnancy after age 34

Name five conditions that increase the risk of developing breast cancer:	1. Lobular/ductal carcinoma in situ (LCIS/DCIS) 2. Atypical hyperplasia 3. BRCA I/II gene positive 4. Sclerosing adenitis 5. Cancer in contralateral breast
What is the most common site of breast cancer?	Upper outer breast quadrant
What are the classic signs and symptoms of breast cancer?	Mass, dimple, nipple retraction, nipple discharge, rash, local edema, and enlarged axillary lymph nodes
Name two imaging tools used to detect breast cancer:	1. Mammography 2. Ultrasound (best for women <30 y/o with fibrous breast tissue)
What findings on mammography are suspicious for malignancy?	Stellate or spiculated mass and microcalcifications
What is the diagnostic evaluation of a nonpalpable, suspicious lesion on mammography?	Stereotactic or needle localized excisional biopsy

Name the breast disease associated with the following statements:

Most common breast malignancy	Ductal carcinoma (90%)
Most common tumor in young women	Fibroadenoma (benign)
Peau d'orange (edema of the dermis) appearance	Inflammatory carcinoma
Most common cause of bloody nipple discharge	Intraductal papilloma
Tumor cells invade epidermal layer of skin near the nipple	Paget's disease of breast
Increased risk of CA in *same* breast	DCIS (premalignant)
Increased risk of CA in *either* breast	LCIS (premalignant)
Solid, mobile, and well-circumscribed round breast mass	Fibroadenoma (benign)
Breast tenderness with menstrual cycle; cysts and nodules	Fibrocystic disease (benign)
Superficial infection of breast; usually caused by *Staphylococcus aureus*; associated with breast feeding	Mastitis

Name the treatment for each of the following breast diseases:

Fibroadenoma	Observation ± biopsy
Fibrocystic disease	Vitamin E and NSAIDs (if cysts present → aspiration; if bloody aspirate → biopsy)
Mastitis	Continue breast feeding; antibiotics
DCIS	Lumpectomy plus x-ray therapy (XRT) or total simple mastectomy
LCIS	Close follow-up (f/u) or *bilateral* simple mastectomy in high-risk patients
Invasive carcinoma	Lumpectomy plus x-ray XRT or modified radical mastectomy (both ± chemotherapy); axillary lymph node dissection and sentinel lymph node biopsy

Name two potential complications of modified radical mastectomy:

1. Arm lymphedema
2. Injury to nerves

What are the major side effects of tamoxifen?

Endometrial cancer and deep venous thrombosis (DVT)

What are the screening recommendations for breast cancer prevention?

1. Monthly self-breast examinations
2. Annual clinical breast examinations after age 40
3. Mammography every 1-2 years after age 40, then annual mammograms after age 50

VASCULAR SURGERY

What are the two major risk factors for peripheral vascular disease (PVD)?

1. Smoking
2. Diabetes mellitus (DM)

Name two common presenting symptoms of PVD:

1. Intermittent claudication
2. Ischemic rest pain

What are the signs of PVD?

Absent pulses, trophic skin changes (shiny skin, loss of hair, thickened toenails), dependent rubor, muscular atrophy, and necrotic tissue (gangrene)

On examination, how can one differentiate between a foot ulcer caused by ischemia versus venous stasis?

Ischemic foot ulcers commonly occur on the toes or feet, but ulcers caused by venous stasis commonly occur on the medial malleolus.

What are the symptoms of claudication?	Reproducible pain in the lower extremities (usually calf muscles) exacerbated by walking and relieved by rest
Is claudication limb-threatening?	No (only 5% will lose the affected limb in 5 years)
Define ischemic rest pain:	Severe foot pain at rest, usually in the distal foot and arch, caused by PVD
What simple maneuver may bring some relief to patients with ischemic rest pain?	Placing foot in dependent position (eg, over side of bed)
What does ischemic rest pain signify?	Limb-threatening condition (85% of patients will lose the affected limb in 5 years)
What is the name of the triad that includes impotence, buttock claudication, and gluteus muscle atrophy?	Leriche syndrome (caused by aortoiliac occlusive disease)
What is the gold standard for the diagnosis of PVD?	Arteriogram (always required preoperatively)
What conservative measures are commonly taken in the management of a patient with PVD?	Smoking cessation, exercise, and aspirin ± clopidogrel
What are the interventional treatment options for PVD?	1. Percutaneous transluminal angioplasty (PTA)—best for focal, short disease of proximal vessels 2. Surgical revascularization 3. Amputation
What are the surgical indications for PVD?	Rest pain, tissue loss, and incapacitating claudication
What are the "six P's" of acute arterial occlusion?	Pain, Pallor, Pulselessness, Paralysis, Poikilothermia, and Paresthesias
What is the most common cause of acute arterial occlusion?	Embolization (85% are caused by thrombi formed in the heart)
What are the treatment options for acute arterial occlusion?	1. Surgical embolectomy 2. Surgical bypass 3. Thrombolytic therapy

What medication must be started in every patient with suspected arterial occlusion?	Heparin
What are the signs and symptoms of compartment syndrome?	Reperfusion injury causing calf pain (especially on passive stretch), tenderness, paralysis, and paresthesias **Note:** pulses may still be present in affected compartment.
What is the definitive treatment for compartment syndrome?	Emergent fasciotomy
Name five risk factors for development of an abdominal aortic aneurysm (AAA):	1. Atherosclerosis 2. Smoking 3. Hypertension 4. Age >60 5. Male gender (M/F: 4/1)
Where is the most common site of an AAA?	Infrarenal
State the risk of rupture annually of an AAA with each of the following diameters:	
<5 cm	4% (9% in 5 years)
Between 5 and 7 cm	7% (35% in 5 years)
>7 cm	20% (75% in 5 years)
What are the indications for surgery in a patient with an AAA?	AAA >5 cm, growth of AAA >4 mm/y, or patient is symptomatic
What is the classic clinical triad of a ruptured AAA?	1. Abdominal pain 2. Hypotension 3. Pulsatile abdominal mass
What is the treatment for a ruptured AAA?	Emergent operation (50% surgical mortality rate)
What are the common postoperative complications in a patient after an AAA repair?	MI (#1 cause of postoperative death), colonic ischemia, anterior spinal syndrome (caused by occlusion of the artery of Adamkiewicz), and acute renal failure

ORTHOPEDICS

For each description, name the
associated orthopedic injury and
its treatment:

Fx of the fifth metacarpal resulting
from closed fist striking a hard
object

Boxer Fx

Tx: closed reduction (CR) and ulnar
splint (pinning for excess angulation)

Note: if skin is broken → debridement
and ABx for presumed human oral
pathogen infection

Most commonly fractured carpal
bone; tenderness in anatomical
snuffbox

Scaphoid Fx

Tx: thumb spica cast

Note: radiographs may be normal up to
2 weeks; ↑ risk for avascular necrosis
(AVN) and nonunion.

Most common Fx of wrist; fall on
outstretched hand (FOOSH) → Fx of
distal radius with dorsal
displacement of distal fragment

Colles Fx

Tx: CR and cast immobilization

Ulnar diaphyseal Fx and dislocation
of radial head

Monteggia Fx (aka "nightstick Fx")

Tx: CR of radial head and open reduction,
internal fixation (ORIF) of ulna

Radial head subluxation; occurs
after being forcefully pulled by the
hand

Nursemaid elbow

Tx: manual reduction (supinate at 90°
elbow flexion)

Radial nerve palsy resulting from
direct trauma to upper arm

Humerus Fx

Tx: hanging arm cast; functional bracing

Radial shaft Fx with dislocation
of distal radioulnar joint

Galeazzi Fx

Tx: ORIF and casting of arm in supination

Most common shoulder dislocation
(95%); due to subcoracoid dislocation

Anterior shoulder dislocation

Tx: CR, sling (2-6 weeks), intense
rehabilitation

Most common Fx in school-age
children; may threaten the brachial
artery

Supracondylar Fx of humerus

Tx: CR and percutaneous pinning

Note: ↑ risk of Volkmann's ischemic
contracture of forearm

Most frequently fractured long bone
in kids; sometimes related to birth
trauma

Clavicular Fx (commonly middle third)

Tx: sling

Pain/tenderness over anterior humeral head resulting from impingement; ⊕ Neer's sign	Rotator cuff injury Tx: NSAIDs; steroid injection; surgery if refractory to steroids
Most common type of hip dislocation; severe trauma (*dashboard injury*) → internally rotated, flexed, and adducted hip	Posterior hip dislocation Tx: **orthopedic emergency**: reduction under sedation; f/u with serial imaging for 2 years (↑ risk of AVN)
Fx associated with falls in osteoporotic women and ↑ risk of AVN and DVT → shortened, externally rotated leg	Femoral neck Fx Tx: ORIF and parallel pinning or hemiarthroplasty; anticoagulate to ↓ risk of DVT
Fx most commonly associated with fat emboli syndrome (dyspnea, hypoxia, confusion, and scleral petechiae)	Fx of the femur Tx: intramedullary nailing of femur
Lower extremity Fx after landing on foot from large vertical drop; part of "lover's triad" (with lumbar compression Fx and forearm Fx)	Calcaneal Fx Tx: ORIF
Most common type of ankle sprain (90%); results from ankle plantar-flexion	Lateral sprain Tx: **RICE: R**est, **I**ce, Compression, Elevation (to ↓ swelling)
Extreme inversion of the foot → Fx of fibula and avulsion at base of the fifth metatarsal	Jones Fx Tx: immobilization without weight bearing
Extreme eversion of the foot → Fx of fibula and avulsion of the medial malleolus	Pott's Fx Tx: ORIF

ABDOMINAL PAIN

State the most common causes of abdominal pain in each of the following locations:	
Right lower quadrant	1. Appendicitis 2. Gynecologic causes: ovarian cyst, PID, ectopic pregnancy, etc 3. Inflammatory bowel disease-Crohn's disease >> UC 4. Meckel's diverticulitis 5. Intussusception

Left lower quadrant	1. Diverticulitis
	2. Gynecologic causes (same as RLQ pain)
	3. Obstructing mass (eg, colon CA)
	4. Constipation
	5. Sigmoid volvulus (may be generalized)
Right upper quadrant	1. Cholecystitis
	2. Choledocholithiasis/cholelithiasis
	3. Cholangitis
	4. Hepatitis
	5. Hepatic tumor (commonly hepatoma)
	6. Right-sided pneumonia
Epigastrium	1. Gastric or duodenal ulcer
	2. Gastritis/gastroenteritis
	3. Pancreatitis
	4. MI
	Note: peritonitis, SBO, mesenteric ischemia, pneumonia, MI, and gastroenteritis may present with pain in any abdominal location.

MAKE THE DIAGNOSIS

21 y/o male presents with hematemesis after ingestion of aspirin and seven shots of whiskey; physical examination (PE): diaphoretic, ↑ HR, epigastric tenderness; EGD: edematous, friable reddened gastric mucosa

Acute gastritis

A patient with h/o PUD presents with melena; PE: ↑ HR, diaphoretic, epigastric abdominal pain; w/u: NGT aspirate is bloody; EGD: visible bleeding vessel distal to the pylorus

Bleeding duodenal ulcer

A patient with h/o multiple abdominal surgeries presents with crampy abdominal pain, N/V, and ↓ bowel movements; PE: hyperactive bowel sounds, abdominal distension; AXR: dilated small bowel loops, absent colonic gas, and multiple air-fluid levels

SBO

40 y/o G4P4 obese woman presents with constant RUQ pain radiating to right scapula with associated N/V; PE: fever, respiratory pause induced by RUQ palpation, and a painful palpable gallbladder; w/u: ↑ WBC, ↑ alkaline phosphatase (ALP); US: thickened gallbladder wall, pericholecystic fluid with gallstones present

Acute cholecystitis

39 y/o male presents with dull, steady epigastric pain radiating to the back after an alcohol binge, N/V; PE: fever, ↑ BP, epigastric tenderness, guarding, and distension; w/u: ↑↑ amylase/lipase, ↑ WBC; AXR: sentinel loop, colon cutoff

Acute pancreatitis

65 y/o black male with h/o smoking presents with anorexia, weight loss, pruritus, and painless jaundice; PE: palpable nontender distended gallbladder, migratory thrombophlebitis; w/u: ↑ direct bilirubin, ALP, CEA, and CA 19-9; Abd CT: mass in head of pancreas

Pancreatic adenocarcinoma

60 y/o black male with h/o GERD presents with weight loss and dysphagia; EGD: partially obstructing mass near GE junction

Esophageal adenocarcinoma

61 y/o white female presents with right-sided breast mass; PE: breast dimpling, nipple retraction; w/u: mammography: irregular spiculated mass with calcifications in upper outer quadrant

Breast cancer

24 y/o female presents with a breast mass; PE: solid, mobile, well-circumscribed rubbery breast mass; US: circumscribed, homogeneous, oval-shaped, hypoechoic mass

Fibroadenoma

65 y/o presents with severe worsening LLQ pain, N/V, and diarrhea; PE: fever, LLQ tenderness, local guarding and rebound tenderness; w/u: ↑ WBC; Abd CT: edematous colonic wall with localized fluid collection

Diverticulitis

30 y/o female presents with periumbilical pain which has now migrated to the RLQ followed by anorexia, N/V; PE: low-grade fever, local RLQ guarding, rebound tenderness, RLQ tenderness upon LLQ palpation; w/u: urine pregnancy test (UPT) negative, ↑ WBC with left shift

Appendicitis

80 y/o white male smoker with h/o CAD presents with abrupt onset of severe abdominal and back pain; PE: ↓ BP, pulsatile abdominal mass

Abdominal aortic aneurysm

55 y/o presents with colicky abdominal pain, small-caliber stools, and occasional melena; PE: cachexia, abdominal discomfort, guaiac ⊕; colonoscopy: obstructing mass seen in ascending colon

Right-sided colon carcinoma

80 y/o woman presents with halitosis, dysphagia, and regurgitation of undigested foods; w/u: barium swallow shows posterior midline pouch >2 cm in diameter arising just above the cricopharyngeus muscle

Zenker diverticulum

55 y/o Asian female with h/o hepatitis B virus (HBV) presents with dull RUQ pain; PE: weight loss, painful hepatomegaly, ascites, and jaundice; w/u: ↑ alanine transaminase/aspartate transaminase (ALT/AST), ↑ α-fetoprotein; Abd CT: mass seen in right lobe of liver

Hepatocellular carcinoma

55 y/o with h/o choledocholithiasis presents with fever, chills, and RUQ pain; PE: jaundice; w/u: ↑ WBC, bilirubin, and ALP; US: stone in common bile duct

Cholangitis

A patient presents to ED after motor vehicle accident (MVA) with LUQ abdominal pain and left shoulder tenderness; PE: guarding, rebound tenderness, ↓ BP, ↑ HR; US: presence of intra-abdominal fluid

Splenic laceration

43 y/o male presents with epigastric pain, diarrhea, and recurrent peptic ulcers; PE: epigastric tenderness; w/u: ↑ fasting gastrin levels, paradoxic ↑ in gastrin with secretin challenge; octreotide scan: detect lesion in pancreas

Zollinger-Ellison syndrome

A trauma patient presents to the ED after MVA with right-sided pleuritic chest pain, dyspnea, and tachypnea; PE: ↓ BP, ⊕ JVD, unilateral absence of breath sounds, hyperresonance on right side, and tracheal deviation away from right side

Tension pneumothorax

71 y/o with h/o atrial fibrillation presents with acute onset abdominal pain and bloody diarrhea; PE: writhing in pain, irregularly irregular heart rhythm, no peritoneal signs; w/u: arteriogram shows lack of visualization of the SMA and its branches

Acute mesenteric ischemia

72 y/o presents with recurrent, low-grade, painless hematochezia; PE: guaiac ⊕ stool; colonoscopy: slightly raised, discrete, scalloped lesion with visible draining vein in right colon

Angiodysplasia

73 y/o smoker with h/o atrial fibrillation and DM presents with acute onset of pain and numbness in left leg; PE: cool, pulseless left leg; w/u: arteriogram reveals complete occlusion of common femoral artery

Acute arterial occlusion

63 y/o Japanese male with h/o atrophic gastritis presents with weight loss, indigestion, epigastric pain, and vomiting; PE: supraclavicular lymph node; w/u: anemia, ⊕ fecal occult blood

Gastric carcinoma

48 y/o with chronic watery diarrhea, hot flashes, and facial redness; PE: shows II/VI right-sided ejection murmur; w/u: ↑ 5-HIAA in urine

Carcinoid syndrome

40 y/o presents with dysphagia, regurgitation, and weight loss; w/u: barium swallow demonstrates dilated esophagus with distal narrowing (*bird beak*)

Achalasia

16 y/o with strong FH of colorectal CA presents with rectal bleeding and abdominal pain; w/u: anemia; flexible sigmoidoscopy: >100 adenomatous polyps visualized

Familial adenomatous polyposis (FAP)

70 y/o male smoker with h/o unintentional 10-lb weight loss presents with dysphagia that started with solids and progressed to liquids; EGD with biopsy: abnormality in upper one-third of esophagus

Esophageal squamous cell carcinoma

40 y/o obese female presenting with RUQ pain, pruritus, dark urine, and clay-colored stools; PE: fever, jaundice, and cutaneous xanthomas; w/u: ↑ ALP and bilirubin

Biliary tract obstruction

35 y/o male presents with sudden, severe onset of abdominal pain radiating to back; PE: appears toxic with peritoneal signs; CXR: free air under the diaphragm

Perforated ulcer

63 y/o male smoker with h/o cardiac bypass surgery presents with pain in both legs exacerbated by walking and relieved with rest; PE: tissue breakdown and ↓ hair growth over distal foot, absent pulses; w/u: ankle-branchial index (ABI) <0.4; Doppler US: arterial stenosis

Peripheral vascular disease (PVD)

36 y/o female who recently completed a course of ABx for a UTI last week presents with watery diarrhea and abdominal cramps; PE: fever and lower abdominal tenderness; w/u: ↑ WBC

Clostridium difficile colitis

35 y/o obese male presents with burning substernal chest pain 30-90 min after meals and worse with reclining; PE: normal; w/u: barium swallow reveals hiatal hernia

GERD

CHAPTER 3

Neurology

HEADACHE

Name the type of headache (migraine, tension, cluster, or sinus) associated with the following features:

Aspirin, nonsteroidal anti-inflammatory drugs (NSAIDs), sumatriptans, ergot alkaloids, and opiates may be used as abortive therapy.	Migraine
Associated with nausea/vomiting (N/V), photophobia, phonophobia	Migraine
β-Blockers, calcium channel blockers, ergots, antidepressants, and depakote are used for prophylaxis.	Migraine
Classic symptoms include unilateral frontotemporal cephalgia with aura and visual symptoms (eg, scintillating scotoma).	Migraine
Characterized by periods of multiple headaches of the same character alternating with symptom-free intervals	Cluster
Ipsilateral tearing, conjunctival injection, Horner syndrome, and rhinorrhea	Cluster
Pulsatile or throbbing headaches	Migraine
May be precipitated by hormonal factors (eg, oral contraceptive pills [OCPs] or menses) and emotional or metabolic stress	Migraine
History of allergies	Sinus

Localized tenderness over sinsuses	Sinus
Most common type of headache in adults	Tension
Pathophysiology may relate to the effect of serotonin on cephalic blood vessels.	Migraine
Patients often have a family history (FH) of headaches.	Migraine
Symptoms are often eradicated by 100% O_2 by facemask or serotonin agonists (sumatriptan).	Cluster
Unilateral boring periorbital headache worst in the temporo-orbital region	Cluster
Vise-like, tightening bilateral pain associated with photophobia, phonophobia, and neck tightness	Tension
4/1 F/M incidence	Migraine
Approximately 95% of cases are in males.	Cluster

What are the seven red flags (suggesting serious underlying pathology) in the diagnosis of headache?

1. Sudden onset of severe headache
2. Headache beginning after straining, Valsalva, sexual activity, or awakens patient from sleep
3. Headache that is persistent and worsening over a period of weeks or months
4. Headache associated with focal neurologic findings or a change in mental status
5. Headache associated with meningeal signs (including nuchal rigidity, Brudzinski's or Kernig's sign)
6. Headache associated with fever
7. Headache in a patient who has never experienced a headache before

What cause of headache is classically associated with the following:

Young, obese female w/ papilledema, negative CT/MRI	Pseudotumor cerebri (benign intracranial hypertension)
Positive Brudzinski's sign	Meningitis
"Worst headache of life"	Subarachnoid hemorrhage

Inflammatory systemic illness in elderly; symptoms include unilateral headache in temporal region, eye pain, and vision loss	Temporal arteritis (giant cell)
High number of polymorphonuclear cells in CSF	Meningitis (bacterial)
Blood in CSF	Subarachnoid hemorrhage
Large doses of Vitamin A or tetracyclines	Pseudotumor cerebri
Medical emergency treated with steroids	Temporal arteritis
Brief episodes of pain in the fifth cranial nerve distribution	Trigeminal neuralgia
Initial treatment options include acetazolamide and diuretics	Pseudotumor cerebri
Polymyalgia rheumatica	Temporal arteritis
What are the common situations in which a lumbar puncture (LP) is contraindicated?	Acute head trauma or signs/symptoms of intracranial hypertension—in these settings, a lumbar puncture should be performed only **after** a negative head CT or MRI.
What is the risk of performing an LP in the setting of acute head trauma?	Uncal herniation and death

SEIZURES

Name the type of seizure associated with the following clinical findings:	
Brief lapses of consciousness with or without rapid eye blinking, slight head, and limb jerking in a child	Absence seizure
First line of therapy may include valproate, phenytoin, carbamazepine, phenobarbital, or newer agents (levetiracetam, oxcarbazepine, lamotrigine)	Tonic-clonic seizure
Sudden, brief muscle contractions; first line of therapy includes valproate and clonazepam	Myoclonic seizures
Commonly mistaken as daydreaming in a young child	Absence seizure

First line of therapy includes ethosuximide and valproate.	Absence seizure
Loss of consciousness followed by loss of postural control, a tonic phase of muscle contraction, and clonic phase of limb jerking	Tonic-clonic seizure
Motor, sensory, visual, psychic, or autonomic phenomena with preserved level of consciousness	Simple partial seizure
3-Hz spike-and-wave pattern on EEG	Absence seizure
May be associated with cyanosis and urinary or fecal incontinence; ↑ serum prolactin during postictal period	Tonic-clonic seizure
Motor, sensory, visual, psychic, or autonomic phenomena with preserved level of consciousness	Simple partial seizure
Motor, sensory, visual, psychic, or autonomic phenomena with diminished level of consciousness and/or postictal confusion	Complex partial seizure
Seizure interferes with a single neurologic modality (motor, sensory, or autonomic function) but does not cause loss of consciousness.	Simple partial seizure
Seizure commonly involves the temporal lobe.	Complex partial seizure
Lack of postictal state	Absence seizure
Presents in infancy w/ sudden extensor/flexor trunk movements; psychomotor retardation; and disorganized high-voltage slow waves, spikes, and sharp waves on EEG	West syndrome (infantile spasms)
Tonic-clonic, generalized seizure occurring in children (6 months to 5 years) caused by fever	Febrile seizure
What is the treatment for febrile seizures?	Acetaminophen (no specific seizure treatment is indicated)
Do most children with febrile seizures go on to develop epilepsy?	No—the risk is barely higher than in the general population.

What are the causes of secondary
seizures?

1. CNS infection
2. Trauma
3. Stroke
4. Drug withdrawal (eg, ethyl alcohol
   (EtOH), barbiturates,
   benzodiazepines, anticonvulsants)
5. Toxins
6. Metabolic (hypoxia, hypoglycemia,
   hyponatremia)
7. Mass effect (from tumor or
   hemorrhage)
8. Cerebral edema (malignant HTN,
   eclampsia)

What is the treatment for status
epilepticus?

1. ABC (airway, breathing, circulation)
2. Roll patient on side to prevent
   aspiration
3. IV diazepam or lorazepam and/or
   phenytoin

CEREBRAL VASCULATURE

What are the two main classifications
of stroke and what is their relative
incidence?

1. Ischemic: >85% of cases
2. Hemorrhagic: <15% of cases

What are the most common causes of
ischemic stroke?

1. Atherosclerotic complications
2. Atrial fibrillation (emboli from clot
   formation)
3. Endocarditis (septic emboli)
4. Sickle cell disease

Describe the artery that has been
occluded in each of the following
stroke syndromes:

Paresis and sensory loss of
contralateral lower extremity

Anterior cerebral artery (ACA)

Hemiparesis, contralateral
hemisensory loss, homonymous
hemianopsia, aphasia

Middle cerebral artery (MCA) supplying
the dominant hemisphere

Altered mental status, memory
deficits, hemisensory loss,
homonymous hemianopsia with
macular sparing

Posterior cerebral artery (PCA)

Amaurosis fugax

Ophthalmic artery

Vertigo, cranial nerve (CN) palsies, impaired level of consciousness, dysarthria	Basilar artery
1. Ataxia 2. Nystagmus 3. Paresis of conjugate gaze 4. Horner syndrome 5. Contralateral decreased pain/temp in face and body 6. Decreased proprioception in LE>UE 7. Dizziness 8. N/V	Superior cerebellar artery (lateral medullary syndrome)
Urinary incontinence, suck and grasp reflexes	MCA or ACA supplying the frontal lobe
1. Ipsilateral nystagmus 2. Facial paralysis 3. Conjugate gaze paralysis 4. Deafness 5. Tinnitus 6. Ataxia 7. Decreased facial sensation 8. Contralateral decreased pain and temp 9. N/V, vertigo	Anterior inferior cerebellar artery
1. Ipsilateral loss of pain and temp in face 2. Contralateral loss of pain and temp in body 3. Ipsilateral laryngeal/pharyngeal paralysis 4. Ipsilateral Horner syndrome 5. Vertigo 6. Ipsilateral ataxia 7. Nausea	Posterior inferior cerebellar artery (Wallenberg syndrome)
Wernicke aphasia (fluent speech without meaning; poor comprehension and word repetition)	Dominant inferior MCA
Broca aphasia (nonfluent speech with poor repetition and normal comprehension)	Superior dominant MCA
What is the most common site for ischemic/embolic stroke?	MCA
What is the most common source of emboli that result in stroke?	Carotid atheroma

Name the term used to describe the infarction of white matter commonly associated with hypertension, diabetes, and carotid atherosclerosis:

Lacunar infarction

Name the term used to describe the infarction of gray matter commonly associated with sustained hypotension:

Watershed infarction (occurs at the margin of arterial territories)

What is the peak period for cerebral edema after a stroke?

2-5 days

Name three noninvasive, non-pharmacologic interventions for lowering intracranial pressure (ICP) that can be used in the setting of stroke or trauma:

1. Elevate the head of the bed at least 30° (maximize venous drainage).
2. Maintain normothermia.
3. Maintain $P_{CO_2} \leq 35$.

Name six medical or surgical interventions for lowering ICP that can be used in the setting of stroke or trauma:

1. Light sedation (ie, benzodiazepines, narcotics, propofol)
2. Osmotic diuresis (mannitol, hypertonic saline)
3. Cerebrospinal fluid (CSF) diversion (ventriculostomy)
4. Chemical paralysis (non-depolarizing muscle relaxants)
5. Barbiturate coma
6. Decompressive craniectomy

Name the term used to describe a neurologic deficit caused by ischemia that resolves within 24 h:

Transient ischemic attack (TIA)

What is the primary radiologic study necessary in the workup (w/u) of stroke?

Computed tomographic (CT) scan of the head **without contrast**

What radiologic study may be useful in determining the etiology of an ischemic stoke?

Cerebral angiography

What radiologic study can provide useful information about the anatomy of a stroke if angiography is contraindicated?

Magnetic resonance angiography (MRA)

What oral medications have been shown to improve outcome in patients with acute ischemic stroke?

Aspirin, clopidogrel, ticlopidine, and Aggrenox

What type of therapy is indicated in a patient at risk for cardioembolic stroke?

Anticoagulation with heparin followed by Coumadin

What medical intervention has been shown to improve outcome in embolic stroke when administered within 3 h?

Tissue plasminogen activator (tPA)

What surgical intervention is indicated for patients with symptomatic carotid stenosis causing >70% compromise of the carotid lumen?

Carotid endarterectomy

What primary preventative measures are recommended in a patient at risk for ischemic stroke?

Smoking cessation, antihypertensive therapy, glycemic control in diabetics, and cholesterol lowering therapy

INTRACRANIAL HEMORRHAGE

Name the type of intracranial hemorrhage associated with the following features:

Associated with cerebral arteriovenous malformations

Subarachnoid and intraparenchymal hemorrhage

Commonly caused by ruptured berry aneurysm; classically presents as "the worst headache of my life"

Subarachnoid hemorrhage

Commonly presents with headache and lethargy in a patient with focal motor and sensory defects

Intraparenchymal hemorrhage

Hematoma following the contour of a cerebral hemisphere on CT; due to laceration of bridging cerebral veins

Subdural hematoma

Lens-shaped hematoma on CT scan; due to laceration of middle meningeal artery due to fracture of the temporal bone

Epidural hematoma

Lumbar puncture (LP) must be performed in a patient with suspected intracranial hemorrhage even if CT scan is negative.

Subarachnoid hemorrhage

Lucid interval followed by rapid decline in mental status

Epidural hematoma

May present with meningeal signs, CN palsies, seizures, and focal neurologic signs; bloody or xanthochromic CSF on LP

Subarachnoid hemorrhage (secondary to ruptured aneurysm)

Most common type of intracranial hemorrhage from trauma

Subdural hematoma (commonly seen in alcoholics and the elderly)

Treated with emergent neurosurgical evacuation	Epidural hematoma (and subdural hematoma >1 cm or with midline shift)
Type of intracranial hemorrhage seen in patients with long-standing, poorly controlled hypertension	Intraparenchymal hemorrhage
What is the most common cause of subarachnoid hemorrhage?	Trauma
What is the most common cause of subarachnoid hemorrhage in a patient with a negative cerebral angiogram?	Perimesencephalic hemorrhage (due to rupture of perimesencephalic veins)
Name a vascular complication of subarachnoid hemorrhage that may cause cerebral ischemia:	Vasospasm (peak incidence 6-8 days after hemorrhage)
Name four connective tissue disorders associated with an increased risk of cerebral aneurysms:	1. Ehlers-Danlos syndrome 2. Polycystic kidney disease 3. Marfan's syndrome 4. Coarctation of the Aorta
Name the most common cause of subarachnoid hemorrhage in IV drug users:	Ruptured mycotic aneurysms (usually in MCA distribution)
What are the two classes of treatment for ruptured cerebral aneurysms?	1. Surgical aneursym clipping 2. Endovascular aneurysm embolization
Name the disorder characterized by recurrent ischemic or hemorrhagic strokes due to progressive idiopathic internal carotid artery stenosis:	Moyamoya disease
What is the characteristic finding of moyamoya disease on cerebral angiogram?	"Puff of smoke": due to formation of collateral cerebral vessels originating from the lenticulostriate and thalamoperforating arteries

BRAIN TUMORS

What are the most common types of brain tumors?	Metastatic tumors
Name the primary brain tumor associated with each of the following clinical or pathologic findings:	
2-year survival rate of 26.5% with standard therapy	Glioblastoma multiforme (GBM)

Benign tumor derived form arachnoid cap cells with well-delineated margins	Meningioma
Epstein-Barr virus (EBV) ⊕ B-cell tumor of the CNS in AIDS patients	CNS lymphoma
Malignant pediatric tumor found exclusively in the posterior fossa	Medulloblastoma (metastasizes through CSF pathways)
Most common pediatric intracranial tumor	Juvenile pilocytic astrocytoma
Most common pediatric supratentorial tumor	Craniopharyngioma
Most common pituitary adenoma	Prolactinoma
Most common pituitary tumor	Pituitary adenoma
Most common primary brain tumor	Glioblastoma multiforme
Multiple lesions at presentation	CNS lymphoma, metastases
Small round blue cell tumor	Medulloblastoma
Tumor arising from ependymal lining of ventricular system that may cause spinal metastases	Ependymoma
Tumor characterized by highly malignant cells bordering necrotic areas	Glioblastoma multiforme
Tumor derived from Rathke pouch	Craniopharyngioma
Tumor of the dorsal root that may grow in a dumbbell configuration through a vertebral foramen	Schwannoma
Tumor which originates from the vestibular division of CN VIII	Schwannoma
Two tumors often presenting with bitemporal hemianopia	1. Pituitary adenoma 2. Craniopharyngioma
Type of tumor that may be found bilaterally in patients with neurofibromatosis II	Acoustic neuroma/Schwannoma
Vascular tumor of cerebellum and retina in patients with von Hippel-Lindau syndrome	Hemangioblastoma
Associated with loss of heterozygosity in chromosomes 1p and 19q that commonly presents with seizures	Oligodendroglioma

Tumor arising near foramen of Monro almost exclusively in patients with tuberous sclerosis	Subependymal giant cell astrocytoma
What are the three modalities used in the treatment of a brain tumor?	1. Surgery 2. Chemotherapy 3. Radiation therapy

CNS INFECTIONS

What are the common symptoms of meningitis?	Fever, headache, neck stiffness, photophobia, and change in mental status
What are the classic signs of meningitis?	Change in mental status and meningeal signs: Kernig's sign, Brudzinski's sign, and nuchal rigidity
What test is necessary to make the diagnosis of meningitis?	CSF analysis (usually obtained by LP)

Name the type of meningitis associated with the following CSF findings:

>1000 polymorphonuclear leukocytes, ↓ glucose, ↑ protein, ↑ CSF pressure	Bacterial meningitis
Increased lymphocytes, minor elevation in protein, normal CSF pressure	Viral meningitis
Increased lymphocytes, minor elevation in protein, dramatically ↓ glucose, elevated CSF pressure	Fungal meningitis
Increased lymphocytes, ↑ protein, ↓ glucose	TB meningitis

Name the most common bacterial pathogens responsible for causing meningitis and the appropriate treatment (Tx) for each of the following demographic groups:

<1 month	Group B strep (commonly *Streptococcus agalactiae*), *Escherichia coli,* and *Listeria* **Empiric Tx:** second-generation cephalosporin and ampicillin **Note:** there are other acceptable empiric antibiotic regimens.

1-3 months	*Streptococcus pneumoniae, Neisseria meningitidis,* and *Haemophilus influenzae* (less common today due to vaccinations)
	Empiric Tx: second-generation cephalosporin, vancomycin, and steroids
3 months to adulthood	*S. pneumoniae* (most common cause of meningitis in adults), *N. meningitidis*
	Tx: third-generation cephalosporin, vancomycin, and steroids
Associated with surgery or trauma to the CNS	*Staphylococcus aureus* **Tx:** Vancomycin and ceftazidime
Adults >60 with chronic illness (including alcoholics)	*S. pneumoniae,* gram-negative bacilli, *Listeria*
	Tx: third-generation cephalosporin, ampicillin, and steroids
Name seven complications of meningitis:	1. Hyponatremia 2. Seizures 3. Subdural effusion (especially with *H. influenzae* meningitis) 4. Cerebral edema 5. Subdural empyema 6. Brain abscess 7. Ventriculitis

Name the type of meningitis or encephalitis classically associated with the following features:

Argyll-Robertson pupil	Syphilis
Frequent cause of encephalitis and intracranial mass lesions in AIDS patients with CD4 count <200	Toxoplasmosis
Latin American immigrant with seizures	Neurocysticercosis (due to *Taenia solium*)
Lymphocytic meningitis, cranial neuropathy, and erythema chronicum migrans	Lyme disease
Maternal exposure to cat feces	Toxoplasmosis
Most common cause of viral encephalitis	Herpes simplex encephalitis
Presents in childhood; elevated gamma globulin and measles antibodies in CSF	Subacute sclerosing panencephalitis

Progressive dementia and myoclonus due to abnormal isoform of prion protein	Creutzfeldt-Jakob disease
Most common type of fungal meningitis; commonly seen in immunosuppressed patients; birds are the host for the pathogen	Cryptococcal meningitis
Paresis and tabes dorsalis (sensory ataxia)	Syphilis
Ring-enhancing lesions associated with focal neurologic deficits	Toxoplasmosis
+ India ink preparation	Crytococcal neoformans
Subacute onset of hemiplegia or visual deficits in an AIDS patient	Progressive multifocal leukoencephalopathy (caused by JC virus)
What CNS infection commonly presents with fever, signs of ↑ ICP, focal neurologic signs, and a ring-enhancing lesion on CT?	Brain abscess
What are the organisms most commonly responsible for brain abscesses?	Anaerobes, gram-positive cocci, gram-negative rods
What is the recommended empiric antibiotic coverage for brain abscess?	Metronidazole and ceftriaxone (or another third-generation cephalosporin)

COGNITIVE DISORDERS

Delirium or dementia?

Waxing and waning level of consciousness	Delirium
Usually a rapid onset	Delirium
Characterized by memory loss	Dementia (think DeMEMtia)
Associated with disturbances in sleep-wake cycle	Delirium
Often irreversible	Dementia
Associated with changes in sensorium (hallucinations and illusions)	Delirium
Inattentiveness	Delirium

Name four major causes of delirium.	**"HIDE"** 1. **H**ypoxia 2. **I**nfection (often UTIs) and ICU psychosis 3. **D**rugs (anticholinergics, opioids, steroids, barbiturates), and withdrawal (especially EtOH) 4. **E**lectrolyte and Endocrine causes
Which two syndromes are classically seen in alcoholics experiencing delirium?	1. Wernicke's encephalopathy 2. Korsakoff's psychosis
What is the primary cause of these two syndromes?	Thiamine deficiency
What are the differences between these two?	Wernicke's (ataxia, ophthalmoplegia, nystagmus, confusion) is the early manifestation and progresses to Korsakoff's (memory loss and confabulation) if left untreated.
List four important steps in the evaluation of a patient with new-onset delirium:	1. Check vitals (including O_2 saturation). 2. Check med list. 3. Check lab values. 4. Check for occult infection.
What is the treatment course for delirium?	Address the underlying cause(s); neuroleptics for agitation
What cognitive disorder is characterized by progressive, global intellectual impairment?	Dementia
What is pseudodementia?	Signs/symptoms of dementia secondary to depression; reversible w/ treatment
What is the most common etiology for dementia?	Dementia of Alzheimer type (DAT)— 70%-80% of cases
Name other common etiologies for dementia:	**"DEMENTIASS"** **D**egenerative diseases (Parkinson, Huntington) **E**ndocrine (thyroid, pituitary, parathyroid) **M**etabolic (electrolytes, glucose, hepatorenal dysfunction, ethanol) **E**xogenous (CO poisoning, drugs, heavy metals)

Neoplastic

Traumatic

Infectious (encephalitis, meningitis, cerebral abscess, syphilis, prions, HIV, Lyme)

Affective disorders (ie, pseudodementia)

Stroke (multi-infarct dementia, ischemia, vasculitis)

Note: vascular causes account for 10% of dementias.

Structural (normal pressure hydrocephalus [NPH])

What treatable causes of dementia must be ruled out?

Vitamin B_{12} deficiency, thyroid/parathyroid disorders, uremia, syphilis, tumors (brain), NPH

Name the type of dementia associated with the following features:

Associated with apolipoprotein E4 (ApoE4), amyloid precursor protein, presenilin, and a_2-macroglobulin genes

Alzheimer

Risk for this type of dementia reduced with appropriate antihypertensive and antiplatelet medications

Vascular or multi-infarct

Cognitive impairment, extrapyramidal signs, and early visual hallucinations

Dementia with Lewy bodies

Insidious onset of difficulties with the activities of daily living and cognitive decline in the absence of other neurologic deficits

Alzheimer

Stepwise dementia in a patient with focal neurologic deficits

Vascular or multi-infarct

Death occurs 5-10 years after the onset of cognitive decline.

Alzheimer

Dementia accompanied by changes in personality, speech disturbance, and extrapyramidal signs

Pick

Triad of chorea, behavioral changes, and dementia

Huntington

Most common cause of dementia; donzepil may be helpful

Alzheimer

Risk factors are identical to those of cerebrovascular disease	Vascular or multi-infarct
Difficulty with vertical gaze	Progressive supranuclear palsy
Frontotemporal atrophy	Pick
Progressive dementia, urinary incontinence, gait disorder	Normal pressure hydrocephalus
Rapidly progressive dementia associated with pyramidal, extrapyramidal, and cerebellar motor decline, myoclonus, and increased startle response	Creutzfeldt-Jakob

MOVEMENT DISORDERS

Name the movement disorder associated with the following features:

Resting tremor, bradykinesia, rigidity, and postural instability → treat with dopamine (DA) replacement therapy	Parkinson disease
Pediatric onset of sudden vocal or motor tics	Tourette syndrome
Chorea, behavioral changes, and dementia	Huntington disease
Postural tremor in the absence of other neurologic deficits	Essential tremor
Paroxysmal unilateral flailing limb movements	Hemiballism (2° to a lesion of the subthalamic nucleus)
Atrophy of the caudate and putamen	Huntington disease
Tremor, ataxia, dysarthria, facial dystonia, parkinsonian signs, cognitive decline secondary to abnormal copper metabolism	Wilson disease
Associated with schizophreniform changes	Huntington disease
Autosomal dominant usually presenting between the ages of 35 and 50	Huntington disease
Autosomal recessive usually presenting between the ages of 5 and 15	Friedreich ataxia

"Shuffling gait" and festination	Parkinson disease
Kayser-Fleischer rings	Wilson disease
Treatment is largely supportive	Huntington disease
Loss of neurons in the substantia nigra	Parkinson disease
Ataxia, areflexia, loss of vibration/ position sense, and cardiomyopathy	Friedreich's ataxia

AMYOTROPHIC LATERAL SCLEROSIS, MULTIPLE SCLEROSIS, AND OTHER DEMYELINATING DISEASES

What are the common symptoms of amyotrophic lateral sclerosis (ALS)?	Asymmetric, slowly progressive limb, bulbar weakness with fasciculations (ie, difficulty swallowing)
What are the classic signs of ALS?	Upper motor neuron (UMN) signs (spasticity, hyperreflexia, clonus, upgoing toes, frontal reflexes) *and* lower motor neuron (LMN) signs (flaccid paralysis, fasciculations)
What are the common EMG abnormalities in ALS?	Denervation potentials in at least three limbs
What is the common presentation of multiple sclerosis (MS)?	"Symptoms separated in time and space"; may include limb weakness, spasticity, optic nerve dysfunction, internuclear ophthalmoplegia, paresthesias, tremor, urinary retention, and vertigo
What are the classic radiologic abnormalities on magnetic resonance imaging (MRI) in a patient with MS?	Periventricular white matter lesions
What are the classic CSF abnormalities in a patient with MS?	Oligoclonal bands and mononuclear pleocytosis
What class of medications can be used during exacerbations?	Steroids
What class of medications can be used to prolong periods of remission?	Immunosuppressants (cyclophosphamide, azathioprine, methotrexate) and immunomodulators (β-interferon and copaxone)

Name the demyelinating disorder
associated with the following clinical
and pathologic features:

Most common demyelinating disorder	MS
Ascending paralysis, facial diplegia, and autonomic dysfunction	Guillain-Barré syndrome
Loss of myelin from globoid and peripheral neurons	Krabbe disease
Charcot's triad (intention tremor, scanning speech, and nystagmus)	MS
Autosomal recessive (AR) disease → progressive paralysis, dementia, ataxia; fatal in early childhood	Metachromatic leukodystrophy
Spinal lesions typically occur in the white matter of the cervical cord	MS
Postviral autoimmune syndrome causing demyelination of peripheral nerves, especially motor fibers	Guillain-Barré syndrome
May present with intranuclear ophthalmoplegia (medial longitudinal fasciculus [MLF] syndrome) or sudden visual loss due to optic neuritis	MS
Albuminocytologic dissociation (↑ CSF protein with normal cell count)	Guillain-Barré syndrome
Rapidly fatal AR disease of childhood associated with globoid bodies in white matter due to deficiency of β-galactocerebrosidase	Krabbe disease
Steroids are contraindicated.	Guillain-Barré syndrome
Genetic disorder causing accumulation of very-long-chain fatty acids resulting in behavioral and a diverse array of changes neurologic deficits	Adrenoleukodystrophy
History of upper respiratory infection (URI) or immunization 1 week prior	Guillain-Barré syndrome

VERTIGO

Name the vertiginous disorder
associated with the following features:

Associated with popping sensation in the middle ear after sneezing, coughing, or straining	Endolymphatic fistula
Caused by head injury, may be associated with hearing loss	Labyrinthine concussion
Episodes of vertigo triggered by sudden changes in position; may be associated with recent trauma	Benign positional paroxysmal vertigo
Progressive hearing loss, episodic vertigo accompanied by nausea and vomiting and sense of fullness in the ear	Ménière disease
Sudden onset of nausea, vomiting, and vertigo; self-limited disorder	Vestibular neuronitis
Vertical nystagmus, weakness, ataxia, CN palsies	Infarction of the vestibular system

NEUROMUSCULAR DISEASE

Name the neuromuscular disease
associated with the following features:

Autoimmune disease usually presenting in women between the ages of 20 and 40; symptoms include ptosis, diplopia, and general muscle fatigability	Myasthenia gravis
X-linked recessive disorder of dystrophin	Duchenne's muscular dystrophy and Becker muscular dystrophy (milder)
Classically seen w/ small cell lung cancer	Eaton-Lambert syndrome
Marked weakness following seizure activity	Todd's postictal paralysis
Autosomal dominant presenting between the ages of 7 and 20; affects the face and shoulder girdle; normal life expectancy	Fascioscapulohumeral dystrophy

Most common type of muscular dystrophy	Duchenne's muscular dystrophy
Begins in adulthood; affects the pelvic and shoulder muscles	Limb-girdle dystrophy
Related to destruction of acetylcholine receptors	Myasthenia gravis
May be associated with thymomas	Myasthenia gravis
Passed from mother to offspring; "ragged red fibers" on muscle biopsy	Mitochondrial myopathies
Muscle weakness, sparing of extraocular muscles; related to impaired release of acetylcholine	Eaton-Lambert syndrome
Autosomal recessive glycogen storage disease that typically presents with cramping after exercise due to lactic acid buildup	McArdle disease
Weakness worsens after repetitive use of muscles, but improves after injection of edrophonium.	Myasthenia gravis
Weakness, myalgia, eosinophilia; history of consuming undercooked pork	Trichinosis
Muscle spasms (including facial muscles), trismus, opisthotonos, autonomic dysfunction	Tetanus
Idiopathic, acute, peripheral facial weakness	Bell's palsy
Autosomal recessive, "floppy infant," delayed milestones, progressive atrophy, dysphagia	Werdnig-Hoffmann (type 1 proximal spinal muscular atrophy)
Weakness worsens after injection of edrophonium; miosis, urinary urgency, and diarrhea may be present.	Organophosphate poisoning
Elevated levels of creatine phosphokinase, pseudohypertrophy of calves, lower than normal IQ	Duchenne's muscular dystrophy
Weakness improves after repetitive muscular stimulation.	Eaton-Lambert syndrome
Autosomal dominant usually presenting between the ages of 20 and 30; inability to relax the grip or release a handshake	Myotonic dystrophy

OPHTHALMOLOGY

Name the ophthalmologic disorder
with the following features:

Acute narrowing of anterior chamber angle associated with prolonged pupillary dilation	Angle closure glaucoma
Treatment includes ophthalmic artery thrombolysis.	Central retinal artery occlusion
Sudden onset of blurred vision, eye pain; examination demonstrates a hard, red, painful eye with nonreactive pupil and increased intraocular pressure (IOP).	Angle closure glaucoma
Most common cause of permanent bilateral visual loss in the United States	Macular degeneration
Gradual increase in IOP with progressive eye pain, colored halos in visual field, and peripheral vision loss	Open angle glaucoma
Sudden, painless unilateral blindness; slowly reactive pupil and cherry red spot on fovea; associated with temporal arteritis	Central retinal artery occlusion
Must be treated emergently by lowering the IOP with acetazolamide; pilocarpine may be used once IOP is lowered.	Angle closure glaucoma
More common in African Americans, age >40 years, and diabetics	Open angle glaucoma
Definitive therapy is laser iridotomy.	Angle closure glaucoma
Loss of night and central vision; examination may show retinal pigment epithelium elevation or hemorrhagic changes.	Macular degeneration
"Blood and thunder" appearance of fundus	Central retinal vein occlusion

Make the diagnosis based upon the
following ophthalmologic signs:

Ptosis, miosis, enophthalmos, anhidrosis	Horner syndrome (interruption of the unilateral sympathetic system)

Unilaterally dilated pupil with slow response to light and accommodation	Adie's pupil (postganglionic parasympathetic lesion)
Small pupils that fail to react to light, but with accommodation preserved	Argyll-Robertson pupil (neurosyphilis)
Pupil is unreactive to direct light, but has intact consensual reflex.	Marcus Gunn pupil (afferent pupillary defect)
Pupil fixed and dilated, ophthalmoplegia, and contralateral hemiparesis	Uncal herniation
Eye is positioned "down and out."	Third cranial nerve lesion
Vertical diplopia	Fourth cranial nerve lesion
Weak abduction of eye	Sixth cranial nerve lesion

Provide the location of the lesion corresponding to the following visual field defect:

Upper quadrant anopsia	Contralateral optic radiations in the temporal lobe
Bitemporal hemianopsia	Optic chiasm
Homonymous hemianopsia	Contralateral optic tract
Monocular blindness	Ipsilateral optic nerve
Lower quadrant anopsia	Contralateral optic radiations in the parietal lobe
Homonymous hemianopsia with ocular sparing	Contralateral occipital lobe

SYNCOPE

Provide the likely etiology of syncope (and related method of evaluation) associated with the following history:

Significant stress or fear	Vasovagal (tilt table)
Patient is on Coumadin.	Cardiac: arrhythmia (ECG)
Prior TIA	Vascular (carotid US)
Progressively worsening headache	Neurologic: intracranial lesion (CT/MRI)
Urinary incontinence	Neurologic: seizure (CT/MRI, EEG)
Diabetic	Endocrine: hypoglycemia (give glucose)

PERIPHERAL NEUROPATHY

What are the common categorical etiologies of peripheral neuropathy?	1. Nutritional: deficiency in vitamins B_1 (thiamine), B_6 (history of isoniazid), B_{12}, and E 2. Metabolic: diabetes, uremia, hypothyroidism 3. Toxins: lead (wrist or food drop) and other heavy metals 4. Medications: isoniazid, aminoglycosides, ethambutol, vincristine 5. Infectious: Lyme disease, HIV, diphtheria 6. Autoimmune: Guillain-Barré, lupus, scleroderma, sarcoidosis, amyloidosis, polyarteritis nodosa 7. Anatomical/trauma: carpal tunnel syndrome (secondary to repetitive activity, acromegally, or hypothyroidism), radial nerve palsy (pressure paralysis), fractures

LOCALIZE THE LESION

Absent reflexes, fasciculations, muscular atrophy	Lower motor neuron
Hyperreflexia, muscular rigidity	Upper motor neuron
Emotional lability, personality changes, apathy, inattention, disinhibition	Frontal lobes
Expressive aphasia	Broca's area (dominant frontal lobe)
Receptive aphasia	Wernicke's area (dominant temporal/parietal lobe)
Inability to repeat with intact speech and comprehension	Arcuate fasciculus
Decreased memory, hyperaggression, hypersexuality	Temporal lobes (amygdala)
Anomia, alexia, agraphia, acalculia	Dominant parietal lobe

Hemineglect (ignoring one side of the body)	Nondominant parietal lobe
Visual hallucinations	Occipital lobes
Cranial nerve III, IV dysfunction	Midbrain
Cranial nerve V, VI, VII, VIII dysfunction	Pons
Cranial nerve IX, X, XI, XII dysfunction	Medulla
Ataxia, dysarthria, nystagmus, dysmetria, intention tremor	Cerebellum
Protruding tongue deviating to the right side	CN XII (hypoglossal nerve) on the right side
Deafness, tinnitus, and/or vertigo	CN VIII (vestibulocochlear nerve)
Anosmia (inability to smell)	CN I (olfactory nerve)
Absent corneal reflex	CN V (trigeminal nerve)
Absent gag reflex	CN IX (glossopharyngeal nerve) or CN X (vagus nerve)
Difficulty turning head to the left	CN XI (spinal accessory nerve) on the left
Dilated and nonreactive pupil	CN III (oculomotor nerve)
Loss of taste in the anterior two-thirds of the tongue	CN VII (facial nerve)
Loss of taste in the posterior one-third of the tongue	CN IX (glossopharyngeal nerve)
Right shoulder droop	CN XI (spinal accessory nerve) on the right
Unilateral shooting pains in the face (tic doulorueux)	CN V (trigeminal nerve)
Hyperacusis	CN VII (facial nerve)
Hoarseness	CN X (vagus nerve)
Inability to close eyes	CN VII (facial nerve)

MAKE THE DIAGNOSIS

55-y/o male presents with lower extremity weakness and muscle atrophy; physical examination (PE): ⊕ Babinski's sign, fasciculations, upper extremity hyperreflexia, and spasticity

Amyotrophic lateral sclerosis

65-y/o presents with a gradual decline in memory and inability to complete activities of daily living; head CT: marked enlargement of ventricles and diffuse cortical atrophy

Alzheimer disease

65-y/o female with h/o spinal metastases presents with pain radiating down the back of leg, saddle anesthesia, urinary retention; PE: absent ankle jerk reflexes; lumbar CT: vertebral fracture with large bony fragment in lumbar spinal canal

Cauda equina syndrome

63-y/o male with h/o cartoid atherosclerosis presents with aphasia and right-sided weakness; PE: dense right hemiparesis, ⊕ Babinski's on right side

Left MCA cerebrovascular accident

20-y/o presents with nausea, vomiting, and headache 2 h after being hit in the temple with a baseball; patient lost consciousness initially but soon recovered; head CT: lens-shaped, right-sided hyperdense mass adjacent to temporal bone

Epidural hematoma

40-y/o with h/o *Campylobacter* enteritis 1 week ago presents with ascending symmetric muscle weakness; PE: absent reflexes; w/u: CSF shows ↑ protein, normal cellular (albuminocytologic dissociation)

Guillain-Barré syndrome

37-y/o male presents with poor memory, depression, choreiform movements, and hypotonia; FH of a father who died at 45 after worsening tremors and dementia; brain MRI: marked atrophy of the caudate nucleus

Huntington disease

25-y/o with h/o bilateral temporal lobe contusions 1 week ago presents with a sudden increase in appetite, sexual desire, and hyperorality.

Klüver-Bucy syndrome

30-y/o female with insidious onset of diplopia, scanning speech, paresthesias, numbness of right upper extremity, and urinary incontinence; w/u: CSF analysis is ⊕ for oligoclonal bands; MRI shows discrete areas of periventricular demyelination.

MS

65-y/o female with h/o neurofibromatosis type 2 presents with headache, right-sided leg jerking, and worsening mental status; PE: papilledema and right-sided pronator drift; head CT: dural-based, enhancing left-sided baseball-sized tumor

Meningioma

50-y/o with a h/o squamous cell carcinoma of the lung presents with N/V, headache, and diplopia; PE: papilledema, left oculomotor palsy, right pronator drift; brain MRI: multiple round, ring-enhancing, hyperintense cortical, and cerebellar lesions

Metastases to brain

30-y/o female presents with unilateral throbbing headache, nausea, photophobia, and scotoma. Similar symptoms occur monthly at the same time of her menstrual cycle.

Migraine headache

62-y/o with urinary incontinence, loss of short-term memory, and dementia; PE: wide-based gate; head CT: massively dilated ventricular system

Normal pressure hydrocephalus

60-y/o presents with gradual onset of pill-rolling tremor; PE: masked facies, stooped posture, shuffling gait, cogwheel muscle rigidity

Parkinson disease

31-y/o presents with loss of libido, galactorrhea, and irregular menses; PE: bitemporal hemianopia; w/u: negative β-hCG

Prolactinoma (Prolactin-secreting pituitary adenoma)

45-y/o presents with the gradual onset of sharp pain radiating from his buttocks down his leg that began 2 weeks ago while lifting a heavy box; PE: positive straight leg raise

Sciatica (2° to acute herniation of a lumbar disc)

50-y/o with h/o polycystic kidney disease presents with "worst headache of life," photophobia, nausea; PE: meningismus, impaired consciousness, right eye deviates down and out; w/u: CSF is xanthochromic.

Subarachnoid hemorrhage (2° to ruptured berry aneurysm of posterior communicating artery)

32-y/o male with h/o Arnold-Chiari malformation presents with bilateral upper extremity muscle weakness; PE: loss of pain and temperature sensation, ↓ DTR in upper extremities, and scoliosis; spine MRI: central cavitation of the thoracic spinal cord

Syringomyelia

75-y/o alcoholic male on warfarin for h/o atrial fibrillation presents with declining mental status, headache, and papilledema; head CT: crescenteric, hypodense 2-cm fluid collection along convexity of skull

Chronic subdural hematoma

30-y/o female with ⊕ FH for renal cell carcinoma presents with gait disturbance and blurred vision; PE: retinal hemangiomas, nystagmus, cerebellar ataxia, and dysdiadokinesia; brain MRI: two cerebellar cystic lesions

von Hippel-Lindau disease

50-y/o with h/o alcoholism presents with psychosis, bilateral CN VI palsy, and ataxia; brain MRI: mamillary body atrophy, periventricular hyperintensity on T2, and diffuse cortical atrophy

Wernicke's encephalopathy

5-y/o boy born 5 weeks premature by spontaneous vaginal delivery is found to have an IQ of 60. Developmentally, he initially sat at 10 months, said his first word at 18 months and walked at 20 months. On physical examination, he currently walks on his tiptoes with a scissoring gait; his legs are hypertonic bilaterally w/ brisk patellar reflexes and upgoing toes.

Cerebral palsy

50-y/o man w/ history of polycystic kidney disease presents to the ED with a progressively worsening headache, which began acutely while working out at the gym. While in the ED he has had a decrease in level of consciousness.

Subarachnoid hemorrhage (secondary to berry aneurysm)

12-mo/o girl with normal development until about the age of 5 months. Since that age, she has regressed in both coordination and language, as she can no longer walk and is not speaking her first words any longer. Her parents have also noticed that she has developed a peculiar behavior of wringing her hands for long periods of time.

Rett syndrome

55-y/o female presenting with headaches and progressive visual loss. Physical exam reveals optic atrophy in the right eye and papilledema in the left.

Foster-Kennedy syndrome (commonly caused by a frontal meningioma causing elevated intracranial pressure and mass effect on a single optic nerve)

52-y/o man who is 10 days s/p embolization of an anterior communicating aneurysm (following subarachnoid bleed) 10 days ago, now presents to the ED with an acute decline in mental status.

Vasospasm

27-y/o man who is asymptomatic is found to have pigmented hamartomas of the iris and pigmented macules on his torso and upper back. Upon questioning, he mentions that father and brother also have these "dark spots" on their skin.

Neurofibromatosis type I

63-y/o man recently diagnosed with lung cancer presents to the ED with acute onset of seizure activity. His family states that he has been more confused and fatigued lately. Hct is obtained and is normal.

Syndrome of inappropriate secretion of antidiuretic hormone (SIADH)

4-mo/o boy of Ashkenazi descent is brought in to see the pediatrician as his mom is concerned about his development. He no longer lifts his head, is less alert, and startles very easily. Upon physical examination, his doctor notices a bright red macula surrounded by a whitish ring.

Tay-Sachs

2-mo/o boy w/ a 2-day history of fever, nasal discharge, and decreased oral intake. Upon physical examination, he is ill appearing, unresponsive to stimulation, and his anterior fontanelle is open and bulging. Fluid from lumbar puncture reveals increased WBC and protein levels and decreased glucose.

Acute bacterial meningitis (*Streptococcus pneumoniae, Neisseria meningitidis, Haemophilus influenzae*)

65-y/o woman with a 4-month history of progressively worse headache presents for evaluation. A subsequent MRI reveals a mass involving the corpus callosum and both frontal lobes. Biopsy shows a poorly differentiated tumor with pleomorphic cells and nuclear atypia.

Glioblastoma multiforme

61-y/o man presents with a broad-based unsteady gait. He denies vertigo. On physical examination, upper limb coordination is within normal limits, and without tremor. However, he is unable to walk in a straight line, and has nystagmus.

Cerebellar vermis lesion

CHAPTER 4

PSYCHIATRY

Describe the types of disorders that fall under each of the following DSM-IV classifications:

Axis I	Clinical psychiatric disorders
Axis II	Personality disorders and mental retardation
Axis III	Medical conditions
Axis IV	Social and environmental factors
Axis V	Global assessment of functioning (GAF)

MOOD DISORDERS

What is the lifetime incidence of major depressive disorder (MDD)?	Approximately 15%
What is the recurrence rate?	>50%
Name the eight key features of MDD besides depressed mood:	**"SIG E CAPS"** 1. **S**leep changes (insomnia/ hypersomnia) 2. **I**nability to experience pleasure, Interest ↓ 3. **G**uilt or feelings of worthlessness 4. **E**nergy ↓ (fatigue) 5. **C**oncentration ↓, indecisiveness ↑ 6. **A**ppetite disturbance with weight change (>5% body weight in 1 month) 7. **P**sychomotor changes (agitation or retardation) 8. **S**uicidal ideations
What features are required to make the diagnosis for MDD?	**Two episodes** of sustained, distinct depressed mood (and at least four symptoms from the previous answer) for **2 weeks**, separated by **2 months**

195

What is in the differential diagnosis for a depressive disorder (d/o)?	MDD, bipolar d/o, dysthymia, cyclothymia, secondary mood d/o, dementia, schizoaffective d/o, d/o not otherwise specified (NOS), and bereavement (<2 months)
Name two types of secondary mood disorders:	1. Mood d/o due to medical condition (eg, endocrinopathies, cancer, CNS infections) 2. Substance-induced mood d/o (ie, steroids, reserpine, α-interferon ethanol, benzodiazepines) **Note:** can be due to intoxication or withdrawal

Depression or bereavement?

Mood fluctuates	Bereavement
Pervasive low self-esteem	Depression
Usually not suicidal	Bereavement
May have sustained psychotic symptoms	Depression
Symptoms improve with time (usually gone by 6 months)	Bereavement
Often open to social support	Bereavement

Name four sleep changes associated with MDD:	1. ↑ sleep latency 2. Early morning waking 3. ↓ stages 3 and 4 sleep 4. ↓ rapid eye movement (REM) latency and REM occurs earlier in the night
What type of depression, more common in children, is characterized by mood lability and rejection sensitivity?	Atypical depression
What are some common predisposing factors for MDD?	Early parental loss, psychiatric or medical illness, and substance abuse
What class of drugs is commonly used first in the treatment of MDD?	Selective serotonin reuptake inhibitors (SSRIs)
Name two other classes of medication used for MDD:	1. Tricyclic antidepressants (TCAs) 2. Monoamine oxidase inhibitors (MAOIs)

How long do antidepressants typically take to have an effect?	4-6 weeks
What is a safe, effective treatment for refractory MDD?	Electroconvulsive therapy (ECT)
What is the suicide rate in MDD?	Approximately 15%-30%
What is the distinctively abnormal, irritable, elevated, expansive mood that lasts >1 week *or* is severely impairing (eg, requiring hospitalization)?	Manic episode
What are the seven key features of mania?	"DIG FAST" (at least three of following for diagnosis): 1. **D**istractibility 2. **I**nsomnia 3. **G**randiosity 4. **F**light of ideas or racing thoughts 5. Psychomotor **A**gitation 6. **S**peech that is pressured or hyperverbal 7. **T**houghtlessness ($\uparrow$ pleasurable activities $\rightarrow$ $\uparrow$ consequences)
What is the diagnosis when less severe manic features (ie, no impairment and absence of psychotic features) are present for at least 4 days?	Hypomania
What is required for the diagnosis of bipolar d/o?	One of more manic episodes (see above) usually accompanied by one or more major depressive episodes
Provide the bipolar classification given the following history of disease:	
Mania and major depression	Type I
Hypomania and major depression	Type II
Four or more mood episodes per year	Rapid cycling
Full symptoms of both mania and depression intermixed or alternating rapidly for at least a week	Mixed

What is the differential diagnosis for bipolar d/o?	Bipolar d/o (I and II), MDD, cyclothymia, schizoaffective d/o, borderline personality d/o, secondary mood d/o
What is the treatment for an acute manic episode?	First, manage agitation (benzos) and control mood (lithium, valproate, carbamazepine); then treat any psychoses.
What is the treatment for bipolar depression?	Mood stabilizing drugs; ECT if refractory

Name the mood d/o associated with the following features:

Chronic d/o >2 years characterized by alternating hypomania and mild depression; absence of euthymia >2 months with no significant impairment	Cyclothymia
Depressed mood for most of the day, for >50% of days, lasting >2 years with at least two signs of depression within last 2 months	Dysthymic d/o **Note:** in kids diagnosis requires irritability and at least 1 year of ↓ mood.
Dysthymia plus MDD	Double depression

SUICIDE AND VIOLENCE

Name the risk factors for suicide:	**"SAD PERSONS"** **S**ex—male (women > attempts; men > actual suicides) **A**ge (bimodal: ↑ 15-24 years and the elderly) **D**epression (or other psychiatric d/o) **P**revious attempts (#1 risk factor) **E**thanol (and other substance abuse) **R**ational thought **S**ickness **O**rganized plan **N**o spouse **S**ocial support lacking
What percentage of those attempting suicide will give warnings of intent?	80% (*ask* about suicidal thoughts, intent, plan)

What is the approach to a patient who voices suicidal intentions? — Emergent inpatient hospitalization

What are three types of family violence?
1. Child abuse
2. Partner abuse
3. Elder abuse

What are some of the risk factors for partner abuse? — Pregnancy, young age, social isolation, child abuse in home

How common is partner abuse in women seeking medical care? — >20%

Name three findings that are suggestive of each type of abuse listed below:

Physical child abuse
1. Healed fractures at different stages
2. Cigarette burns
3. Retinal hemorrhage/detachment

Note: 32% of kids <5 y/o are physically abused.

Sexual child abuse
1. Genital/anal trauma
2. STDs
3. UTIs

Note: 25% of kids <8 y/o are sexually abused.

Elder abuse
1. Evidence of depleted finances
2. Poor hygiene
3. Spiral fractures

PSYCHOTIC DISORDERS

What is term used to describe an impairment in the ability to judge boundary between real and unreal? — Psychosis

Give the appropriate term for each of the following psychotic symptoms:

False belief or wrong judgment held with conviction despite incontrovertible evidence to the contrary — Delusion

False perception of an actual external stimulus — Illusion

Thought d/o whereby ideas are not logically connected to those that occur before or after — Loose association

Misinterpreting others' actions or environmental cues as being directed toward one's self when, in fact, they are not	Idea of reference
Subjective perception of an object or event when no such external stimulus exists	Hallucination
What is the prevalence of schizophrenia?	0.9%-1.2%
What is the risk of schizophrenia in primary relatives of a schizophrenic?	Siblings: 10%; parents of patient: 5.9%; kids of patient: 12.8%
What is the rate of suicide in schizophrenics?	10% at 10 years
What is the typical age of onset for schizophrenia?	Females: 25-35, males: 15-25
What is the differential for schizophrenia?	Schizoaffective d/o, schizophreniform d/o, brief psychotic d/o, delusional d/o, bipolar d/o, personality d/o, drug intoxication or withdrawal, and psychotic d/o due to a medical condition
What are the five main diagnostic criteria for schizophrenia?	1. Delusions 2. Hallucinations 3. Disorganized speech 4. Grossly disorganized or catatonic behavior 5. Negative symptoms
Name the key features of schizophrenia:	Two or more psychotic symptoms for >1 month; impairment of social/occupational functioning; all >6 months
What are the guidelines for hospitalization for schizophrenia?	Hospitalize during psychotic episode if danger to self/others or unable to care for self.
How is schizophrenia managed between psychotic episodes?	Treat antipsychotics and supportive psychotherapy; symptom monitoring
Give three examples of positive symptoms that are characteristic of schizophrenia:	1. Hallucinations 2. Delusions 3. Disorganized thought processes (eg, loose associations)
Positive symptoms respond best to what types of drugs?	Traditional antipsychotics (haloperidol)

Give five examples of negative symptoms that are characteristic of schizophrenia:	**The five A's** 1. **A**ffect flattened 2. **A**logia 3. **A**nhedonia 4. **A**volition 5. Poor **A**ttention
Negative symptoms respond best to what types of drugs?	**A**typical antipsychotics (clozapine, risperidone); atypicals **for four A's**
What factors are associated with a better prognosis?	1. Good premorbid functioning (most important) 2. Acute and late onset 3. Obvious precipitating factors 4. Strong support system 5. Married status 6. Positive symptoms 7. Family history of mood d/o 8. Early and continued treatment (including medication compliance) 9. Female gender 10. Absence of structural brain abnormality
Low-potency traditional antipsychotic agents are more likely to cause what types of side effects?	Anticholinergic, sedation, and hypotension
High-potency traditional antipsychotic agents are more likely to cause what types of side effects?	Neurologic (extrapyramidal symptoms [EPS], dystonia, tardive dyskinesia, and so on)
Name the DSM-IV subtype of schizophrenia associated with the following features:	
Delusions of persecution	Paranoid
Disinhibition; poor organization, personal appearance, and grooming	Disorganized (aka hebephrenic)
One previous schizophrenic episode with attenuated symptoms, but no active positive psychotic symptoms	Residual
Characteristics of more than one subtype	Undifferentiated
Bizarre posturing, mutism, stupor, *or* extreme excitability	Catatonic
Older age of onset, better functioning than other subtypes	Paranoid
Age of onset typically before 25 years	Disorganized

Name the psychotic d/o characterized by the following descriptions:

Psychotic symptoms lasting >1 day, but <1 month (often with obvious precipitating psychosocial stressor)	Brief psychotic d/o
Psychotic symptoms lasting 1-6 months	Schizophreniform d/o
Fixed, nonbizarre delusional system; without other thought disorders or impaired functioning	Delusional d/o
Symptoms of major mood d/o as well as of schizophrenia (with psychotic features occurring before mood disturbance); chronic social and occupational impairment	Schizoaffective d/o
Clouded consciousness, predominantly *visual* hallucinations, often occurring in inpatient setting	Psychotic d/o due to a general medical condition
Social withdrawal without psychosis	Schizoid personality d/o
Odd thought patterns (eg, magical thinking) combined with peculiar behavior, without psychosis	Schizotypal personality d/o
Adopting the delusional system of a psychotic person	Shared psychotic d/o (Folie à deux)

What type of delusional d/o is characterized by the following:

One is conspired against	Persecutory (most common)
One is loved by a famous person	Erotomanic
One possesses great talent	Grandiose
One has a physical abnormality	Somatic
Belief that spouse/lover is unfaithful	Jealous

ANXIETY DISORDERS

What anxiety d/o is characterized by the recurrent, sudden-onset chest pain, palpitations, tachypnea, dizziness, nausea, trembling, and diaphoresis associated with intense fear (and lasts for 10 min)?	Panic d/o

What is the differential diagnosis for panic d/o?	Angina/myocardial infarction (MI), substance-induced anxiety, generalized anxiety d/o, posttraumatic stress disorder (PTSD), and thyroid storm
What additional symptoms that follow these attacks are required to diagnose panic d/o?	Persistent concern about more attacks and worrying about the implications of the panic attacks
What phobia is often associated with panic d/o?	Agoraphobia
Age at onset?	Mid- to late twenties
What medical conditions can be associated with panic d/o?	Mitral valve prolapse, hyperthyroidism, vitamin B_{12} deficiency, hypoglycemia, pheochromocytoma, arrhythmia, and CNS diseases
What anxiety d/o is characterized by marked, persistent fear of an object/situation which results in an unreasonable and excessive response, and thus the stimulus is avoided?	Specific phobia
What is the prevalence of specific phobias?	10%-20% of the population (female >> males)
How does specific phobia differ from social phobia?	Unlike social phobia, specific phobia is a fear directed toward a specific object or situation.
What is the treatment of choice for specific phobias?	Exposure therapy (eg, desensitization, flooding)
What anxiety d/o can occur after a person is subjected to a traumatic event?	PTSD
Name the five major criteria for diagnosing PTSD:	1. Exposure to a traumatic event causing intense fear or horror 2. Reexperiencing the event (in dreams, flashbacks, and so on) 3. Avoiding stimuli related to the trauma and overall emotional "numbing" of responsiveness 4. Symptoms of hyperarousal/hypervigilance 5. Clinically significant impairment
What two traumatic events are *most likely* to cause PTSD in males and females?	**Males:** Rape > combat **Females:** Childhood abuse > rape

What often complicates the treatment of PTSD?	Substance abuse
What is the treatment approach for PTSD?	First, address any underlying substance abuse; SSRIs (fluoxetine) and MAOIs (phenelzine); β-blockers for autonomic symptoms; and behavioral therapy and support groups
What anxiety d/o is characterized by symptoms of PTSD that occur within 4 weeks of the stressor and last <4 weeks?	Acute stress d/o
What anxiety d/o is characterized by excessive worrying for >50% of the days over the past 6 months that causes significant impairment?	Generalized anxiety d/o; prevalence: 4%-9% (females >> males)
What comorbidity is common in a person w/ general anxiety d/o	Depression
What is the treatment of choice for generalized anxiety d/o?	Combined therapy: psychotherapy and medication
What medications are preferred for treating generalized anxiety d/o?	Intermediate-acting benzodiazepines (less addiction, last reasonably long) or buspirone (preferable in those with addiction potential); antidepressants in patients with comorbid depression
What anxiety d/o is characterized by maladaptive behavioral symptoms related to an identifiable stressor, which occurs *within 3 months* of a traumatic incident and results in functional impairment?	Adjustment d/o
What term is used to describe recurrent, intrusive, senseless thoughts, images, and impulses?	Obsessions
What term is used to describe repetitive behaviors driven by the conscious will to respond to an obsession and thereby decrease the anxiety caused by it?	Compulsions
Name three common obsessions:	1. Contamination 2. Symmetry 3. Fear of being harmed (or harming others)

Name three common compulsions:	Three C's of Compulsion
	1. Cleaning
	2. Checking
	3. Counting

Name three ways in which obsessive-compulsive disorder (OCD) differs from obsessive-compulsive personality type:	1. The d/o causes significant distress and impaired functioning.
	2. Patients are aware that their behaviors are unreasonable, but are not able to control them.
	3. The personality type lacks true obsessions/compulsions.

What is the treatment of choice for OCD?	SSRIs (fluvoxamine) or TCAs (clomipramine), and cognitive-behavioral therapy

SOMATOFORM DISORDERS

What somatoform d/o is characterized by multiple, often vague and unrelated, physical complaints leading to excessive medical attention seeking and severely impaired functioning?	Somatization disorder (F/M = 5/1)

Typical age of onset?	Before 30

Predisposing factors?	Genetic predisposition and sexual abuse

What combination of complaints fulfills the diagnostic criteria for somatization d/o?	Complaints of four pain, two GI, one sexual/GU, and one pseudoneurologic symptoms
	Note: cannot be intentional or fake

Treatment for somatization d/o?	Regularly scheduled visits to primary care physician; only order tests when there is evidence of illness; antidepressants for comorbid depression (avoid opiates and benzos)

Name the somatoform d/o characterized by the following descriptions:	
Prolonged preoccupation with concerns of having a serious illness (despite negative medical workups) and exaggerated attention to bodily or mental sensations	Hypochondriasis

Conscious simulation of physical or psychologic illness solely to receive attention from medical personnel	Factitious d/o (Munchausen syndrome) **Note:** technically *not* a somatoform d/o because it is intentional
Intentionally simulating illness for personal gain (usually financial)	Malingering **Note:** also *not* a somatoform d/o; suspect in cases involving litigation
Preoccupation with an imagined physical defect, causing significantly impaired social and occupational functioning	Body dysmorphic disorder (BDD)
Sudden onset of motor/sensory neurologic d/o following a traumatic emotional event	Conversion d/o

EATING DISORDERS

What eating d/o is characterized by refusal to maintain normal body weight and extreme fear of becoming obese, resulting in life-threatening weight loss?	Anorexia nervosa; prevalence = 1% in adolescent females (90% of cases are female)
Name four important features in the patient history that suggest anorexia nervosa:	1. Distorted body image (perceive self as being fat) 2. Intense fear of gaining weight, >15% less than ideal body weight 3. Amenorrhea 4. Excessive exercise
What tests should be included in the workup of anorexia nervosa?	Accurate height/weight measurements, ECG, electrolytes, CBC, total protein, β-hCG, thyroid tests, and psychiatric evaluation
What is the appropriate management of anorexia nervosa?	1. Correct nutritional/electrolyte status 2. Psychotherapy 3. Monitor weight, food/calorie intake, and urine output
When should patients be hospitalized	Severe dehydration, starvation, hypotension, electrolyte problems, hypothermia, risk of suicide
What is the mortality rate in anorexia nervosa?	6%-20%

What eating d/o is characterized by episodes of binge eating associated with emotional distress and accompanied by compensatory behaviors aimed at preventing weight gain?	Bulimia nervosa

Name six compensatory behaviors that patients employ to prevent weight gain from bingeing:

1. Self-induced vomiting
2. Diuretic abuse
3. Laxative abuse
4. Use of appetite suppressants
5. Vigorous exercise
6. Medications intended to speed up the metabolism (eg, thyroid hormone)

Name four important features in the patient history that suggest bulimia nervosa:

1. Distorted body image
2. Relatively normal body weight
3. Avoid eating around others
4. Morbid preoccupation with food/eating that leads to binge eating episodes

Name three physical examination findings that may suggest bulimia nervosa:

1. Bilateral parotid enlargement
2. Periodontal disease or extensive dental erosions
3. Russel's sign

What is Russel's sign?

Scarring and abrasions on the knuckles from repeated self-induced vomiting

What laboratory abnormality is often seen with bulimia nervosa?

Metabolic alkalosis (>50%)—from vomiting

What is the treatment course for bulimia nervosa?

Cognitive-behavioral therapy and SSRIs

What antidepressant is contraindicated in bulimia?

Bupropion (Wellbutrin)—↑ risk of seizures

SUBSTANCE ABUSE

What is the lifetime prevalence of substance abuse/dependence?

~13%

Provide the term used to define the following:

Recurrent, maladaptive pattern of substance use for (12 months despite significant consequences (physical hazard or legal, social, or occupational problems)

Abuse

Characterized by craving, tolerance, and/or withdrawal to substance; loss of control with a preoccupation for obtaining and using the substance	Dependence
Maladaptive behavior that is related to recent ingestion of a substance	Intoxication
Substance-specific syndrome following a decrease or cessation of regular use	Withdrawal
The need to increase the amount of an ingested drug to produce the same degree of intoxication	Tolerance
Not counting tobacco and caffeine, what is the most commonly abused substance in the United States?	Alcohol
What is a short, useful screening tool for alcoholism?	"CAGE" questions Have you felt the need to Cut down? Have you ever felt Annoyed by criticism of your drinking? Have you ever felt Guilty about drinking? Have you ever had an Eye opener?
What is the major complication of alcohol withdrawal and when is it most likely to occur?	Delirium tremens (DTs); peak occurrence is 2-7 days. Note: DTs are a medical emergency.
What is the mortality rate of DTs?	15%-20%
What is the medical management of alcohol withdrawal?	Benzodiazepine taper for symptoms; haloperidol for hallucinations; thiamine, folate, and multivitamin replacement; correct electrolyte abnormalities; eventual group therapy or 12-step program
Name three GI complications of alcoholism:	1. GI bleeding (from ulcers, gastritis, esophageal varices, or Mallory-Weiss tears) 2. Pancreatitis 3. Liver disease
What syndrome of anterograde amnesia, confabulations, ataxia, and nystagmus results from chronic alcoholism?	Wernicke-Korsakoff syndrome

What am I high on?

CNS and respiratory depression, euphoria, pinpoint pupils, nausea, and ↓ GI motility	Opioids (goosebumps → *cold turkey*); inspect for track marks along veins
Psychomotor agitation, dilated pupils, euphoria, ↑ heart rate (HR) and BP, prolonged wakefulness and attention, delusions, ↑ pain threshold	Amphetamines
All of the symptoms listed in the previous two questions, plus tactile hallucinations, angina, and sudden cardiac death	Cocaine
Intense violence, psychosis, and delirium; psychomotor agitation, nystagmus, ataxia; rhabdomyolysis and hyperthermia	Phencyclidine hydrochloride (PCP)
Restlessness, insomnia, flushing, GI disturbance, anxiety, diuresis, cardiac arrhythmia	Caffeine
Delusions, visual hallucinations, postuse flashbacks	Lysergic acid diethylamide (LSD)
Light-headedness, euphoria, disinhibition, hallucinations, ataxia, confusion; breathing problems and facial with chronic use	Inhalants (hydrocarbons, glues, volatile cleaners, etc)
Disinhibition, emotional lability, slurred speech, ataxia, blackouts, coma	Alcohol
Euphoria, heightened sensation, increased appetite, dry mouth, conjunctival injection, apathy	Cannabinoids
Increased muscularity, acne, testicular atrophy; chronic use may cause psychosis and/or depression	Anabolic steroids

What am I coming down from and how is it treated?

Anxiety and "flu-like symptoms" (insomnia, piloerection, fever, rhinorrhea, yawning, ↑ GI motility)	Opioids → naltrexone/naloxone for overdose; methadone for detoxification
Recurrence of sudden-onset, homicidal violence, and psychosis	PCP → antipsychotics and benzodiazepines

Hypersomnolence, fatigue, depression, malaise, severe craving for drug (peaks 2-4 days after last dose)	Cocaine → haloperidol, benzodiazepines, antiemetics, anti-inflammatory (for myalgias); bromocriptine for withdrawal
Postuse "crash" (lethargy, headache, hunger, depression, dysphoric mood, altered sleep)	Amphetamines → similar to cocaine
Tremor, ↑ HR and BP, malaise, nausea, seizures, agitation, delirium	Alcohol → (similar to cocaine)

CHILDHOOD DISORDERS

Name the d/o of childhood described
by each of the following statements:

Repetitive behaviors (in patient <18 y/o) that violate social norms; may exhibit physical aggression, cruelty to animals, vandalism and robbery, along with truancy, cheating, and lying	Conduct d/o **Remember:** predominantly *actions*
Recurrent pattern of negativistic, hostile, and disobedient behavior toward authority figures; loss of temper and defiance (but not theft lying)	Oppositional defiant d/o **Remember:** predominantly *words*
Developmentally inappropriate degrees of inattention, impulsiveness, and hyperactivity at home, in school, and in social situations; present *before age 7*	Attention-deficit hyperactivity disorder (ADHD)
Pervasive developmental disorder (PDD) with stereotyped movements and nonprogressive impairments in social interactions, communication, and behavior	Autism
Progressive syndrome of autism, dementia, ataxia, and purposeless hand movements; associated with hyperammonemia; principally in girls	Rett syndrome
PDD with severe impairment in social skills and repetitive behaviors, leading to impaired social and occupational functioning but without significant delays in language development	Asperger d/o

Excessive anxiety concerning separation from home or from those to whom the child is attached

Separation anxiety d/o

Multiple motor and ≥1 vocal tics that persist at least 1 year. Examples of tics include: grimacing, blinking, echopraxia, coprolalia (33%), and echolalia.

Tourett's d/o (*should also evaluate for ADHD [50%] and OCD [40%]*)

Voluntary or involuntary repeated passage of feces into inappropriate places *after* age 4, not due to a medical condition

Functional encopresis (r/o Hirschsprung's disease)

Voluntary or involuntary repeated voiding of urine into bed or clothes *after* age 5, not due to a medical condition

Functional enuresis (r/o UTI, diabetes, seizures)

IQ ≤70 with impaired adaptive functioning in two or more of the following: communication, self-care, academics, home living, social skills, work

Mental retardation (90% are mildly retarded w/ IQ between 55 and 70)

PERSONALITY DISORDERS

Name four qualities that distinguish a personality d/o from a personality *trait:*

1. Maladaptive
2. Enduring (lifelong)
3. Inflexible
4. Impairs social/occupational functioning

List the three cluster A personality disorders:

"Weird"
1. Paranoid
2. Schizoid
3. Schizotypal

List the four cluster B personality disorders:

"Wild"
1. Histrionic
2. Borderline
3. Antisocial
4. Narcissistic

List the three cluster C personality disorders:

"Worried"
1. Avoidant
2. Obsessive-compulsive
3. Dependent

Name the personality d/o characterized
by each of the following statements:

Social inhibition (but desires relationships), sensitive to rejection, inferiority complex	Avoidant (C)
Peculiar appearance, interpersonal awkwardness, "magical" or odd thought patterns, no psychosis	Schizotypal (A)
Impulsive, unstable mood, chaotic relationships, sense of feeling empty and alone, self-mutilation, females >> males	Borderline (B)
Sense of entitlement, grandiosity, lack empathy for others, insists on special treatment when ill	Narcissistic (B)
Suspicious and distrustful, uses projection as primary defense mechanism	Paranoid (A)
Lacks self-confidence, submissive, and clingy	Dependent (C)
Unable to maintain intimate relationships, extroverted, melodramatic, sexually provocative	Histrionic (B)
Disregards and violates rights of others, criminality, males > females; <18 y/o = conduct d/o	Antisocial (B)
Lifelong pattern of voluntary social withdrawal, no psychosis, shows minimal emotions	Schizoid (A)

MISCELLANEOUS PSYCHIATRIC DISORDERS

Name the dissociative d/o characterized
by each of the following statements:

Presence of two or more distinct personalities that recurrently take control of the person's behavior	Dissociative identity d/o
Sudden travel away from home with confusion and amnesia about identity. Assumption of new identity is common.	Psychogenic fugue
Persistent or recurrent feeling of detachment from one's body or self	Depersonalization d/o

Name the sexual d/o characterized
by each of the following statements:

Deficient or absent sexual fantasies or desire	Hypoactive sexual desire d/o
Involuntary spasm of musculature of vagina which interferes with sexual intercourse	Vaginismus
Revulsion to and avoidance of sexual contact	Sexual aversion d/o
Persistent delay or absence of orgasm following sexual excitement	Orgasmic d/o
Persistent ejaculation with minimal stimulation	Premature ejaculation
Inability to attain or maintain an erection to complete sexual activity	Male erectile d/o (impotence)—20%-50% due to medication or medical condition
Inadequate subjective excitement and lubrication in females	Female sexual arousal d/o
Distress about assigned sex; desire to be or insisting one is the opposite sex	Gender identity d/o
Recurrent and intense sexual arousal in response to unusual objects or fantasies lasting ≥6 months	Paraphilias

Name the paraphilia:

Observing unsuspecting person	Voyeurism
Cross-dressing	Transvestism
Exposure of one's genitals to strangers	Exhibitionism (M>>F)
Use of inanimate objects (underwear)	Fetishism (M>>F)
Acts of being beaten, humiliated, bound, made to suffer	Sexual masochism
Prepubescent children	Pedophilia
Suffering of victim	Sexual sadism (M>>F)
Rubbing nonconsenting person	Frotteurism

Name the sleep d/o characterized by
each of the following statements:

Disturbance in initiating, maintaining, or feeling rested after sleep	Primary insomnia

Daytime drowsiness with irresistible sleep attacks	Narcolepsy
Prolonged sleep, excessive daytime sleepiness	Primary hypersomnia
Episodes of breathing cessation during sleep accompanied by snoring, gasping, morning headache, daytime sleepiness, inattention; predisposed by obesity	Sleep apnea
Mismatch between environment demands and person's sleep-wake pattern	Circadian rhythm sleep d/o
Agonizing, deep creeping sensations in leg or arm muscles, relieved by moving or massage	Restless leg syndrome
Awaken with scream, intense anxiety (sleep stage 3 to 4); morning amnesia of episode	Sleep terror d/o
Distressing dreams causing repeated awakenings (during REM); may recall detail in the morning	Nightmare d/o
Episode of coordinated movement (eg, walking) with person unresponsive during episode (sleep stage 3 to 4); morning amnesia	Sleep walking d/o

Name the impulse control d/o characterized by each of the following statements:

Episodes of loss of control of aggressive impulses out of proportion to precipitant	Intermittent explosive d/o
Stealing unnecessary or trivial items	Kleptomania
Maladaptive gambling behavior	Pathologic gambling
Intentional fire setting and fascination with fire	Pyromania
Pulling out of one's own hair, resulting in noticeable hair loss	Trichotillomania

PSYCHOPHARMACOLOGY

Antidepressants

For each of the following drugs, provide: (1) the mechanism of action (MOA), (2) indication(s) (IND), and (3) significant side effects and unique toxicity (TOX) (if any):

TCAs (imipramine, clomipramine, amitriptyline, desipramine, nortriptyline, doxepin, amoxapine)

MOA: prevents reuptake of norepinephrine (NE) and 5-hydroxytryptamine (5-HT)

IND: depression, enuresis (imipramine), depression in elderly (nortriptyline), OCD (clomipramine), depression with psychotic features (amoxapine), fibromyalgia

TOX: sedation (desipramine is least sedating), anticholinergic effects, lethal in overdose → respiratory depression, hyperpyrexia, and

TriCs: Cardiac arrhythmia, Convulsions, Coma

SSRIs (fluoxetine, paroxetine, sertraline, citalopram, fluvoxamine, escitalopram)

MOA: selectively blocks reuptake of 5-HT (usually requires 2-3 weeks to take effect)

IND: depression, premenstrual syndrome (flouxetine), OCD (fluvoxamine)

TOX: agitation, insomnia, sexual dysfunction, "Serotonin syndrome" with MAOIs (muscle rigidity, hyperthermia, cardiovascular collapse)

Bupropion

MOA: heterocyclic agent; has weak reuptake blocking effects on serotonin and NE; also affects reuptake of dopamine

IND: depression, smoking cessation; also used in ADHD

TOX: agitation, seizures, insomnia (↓ sexual side effects)

Trazodone

MOA: mainly inhibits serotonin reuptake

IND: depression

TOX: Postural hypotension, sedation, priapism

Venlafaxine	**MOA:** inhibits 5-HT and NE reuptake
	IND: depression, generalized anxiety d/o
	TOX: stimulant effects, minimal effects on P450
Mirtazapine	**MOA:** $5\text{-}HT_2$ receptor antagonist and a_2-antagonist $\rightarrow$ $\uparrow$ NE and 5-HT release
	IND: depression
	TOX: highly Sedating, $\uparrow$ appetite, $\uparrow$ cholesterol, weight gain
MAOIs (TIP: Tranylcypromine, Isocarboxazid, Phenelzine)	**MOA:** nonselective MAOIs
	IND: atypical depressions, anxiety disorders, pain disorders, eating disorders
	TOX: hyperadrenergic crisis with tyramine (cheese, liver, red wine, aged meets) or meperidine ingestion; serotonin syndrome (diarrhea, nausea, headache, tremor, neuromuscular irritability, hyperthermia, HTN, seizures, death) with SSRIs
Lithium	**MOA:** prevents generation of (IP_3) and (DAG) $2°$ messenger systems
	IND: bipolar d/o (prevents and treats acute mania)
	TOX: hypothyroidism, nephrogenic diabetes insipidus (DI), teratogenesis (Ebstein anomaly)

Antipsychotics

What is the name for stereotyped oral-facial movements that occur as a result of long-term antipsychotic use?	Tardive dyskinesia
Describe the chronology of extrapyramidal side effects from neuroleptic medications:	**"Rule of 4s:"** **4** h: acute dystonia, **4** days: akinesia, **4** weeks: akathesia, **4** months: tardive dyskinesia (usually irreversible)
What is the characteristic triad of neuroleptic malignant syndrome (NMS)?	1. Muscle rigidity 2. Autonomic instability 3. Hyperpyrexia
What is the treatment for NMS?	Dantrolene and dopamine agonists

For each of the following drugs,
provide: (1) the mechanism of action
(MOA), (2) indication(s) (IND), and
(3) significant side effects and unique
toxicity (TOX) (if any):

Traditional high-potency antipsychotics (haloperidol, perphenazine, trifluoperazine)

MOA: D_2 dopamine receptor antagonists (also block a_2, muscarinic, and histaminic receptors)

IND: schizophrenia, psychosis (especially positive symptoms)

TOX: ↑ neurologic (eg, extrapyramidal) side effects (SEs), NMS, tardive dyskinesia

Traditional low-potency antipsychotics (chlorpromazine, thioridazine)

MOA: D_2 dopamine receptor antagonists (also block a_2, muscarinic, and histaminic receptors)

IND: schizophrenia, psychosis

TOX: ↓ neurologic SEs, ↑ anticholinergic and endocrine SEs; cardiac conduction defects and retinal pigmentation (thioridazine), corneal and lenticular deposits (chlorpromazine)

Atypical antipsychotics (clozapine, risperidone, olanzapine, quetiapine)

MOA: 5-HT_2 antagonists; D_4 and $D_1 > D_2$ receptor antagonists

IND: schizophrenia, psychosis (especially *negative* symptoms); OCD/anxiety d/o (olanzapine)

TOX: ↓ anticholinergic and EPS, ↑ hematologic SEs; agranulocytosis (clozapine → weekly WBC monitoring)

Name the drug of choice in each of the following clinical settings:

Depression with insomnia; chronic pain

Amitriptyline (Elavil)

OCD

Clomipramine (Anafranil) or fluvoxamine (Luvox)

Depression with anorexia nervosa or bulimia

Desipramine (Norpramin)—stimulates appetite

Depression with psychotic features

Amoxapine (Asendin)

Refractory psychosis with predominantly negative symptoms

Clozapine (Clozaril)

Panic d/o with agoraphobia

Imipramine (Tofranil)

ADHD in children

Methylphenidate (Ritalin, Concerta, Methylin)

Adult ADHD	Bupropion (Wellbutrin, Zyban)
Premenstrual dysmorphic d/o	Fluoxetine (Paxil)
Trichotillomania	Clomipramine (Anafranil)
Intractable hiccups, with nausea and vomiting	Chlorpromazine (Thorazine)
MDD	Fluoxetine (Paxil)
Anxiety in the elderly	Buspirone (BuSpar)—less sedating
Tourette d/o	Pimozide (Orap)
Alcohol withdrawal symptoms	Chlordiazepozide (Librium)
Smoking cessation	Bupropion (Wellbutrin, Zyban)
Generalized anxiety d/o	Venlafexine (Effexor) or buspirone (Buspar)
Enuresis	Imipramine (Tofranil)
Used to decrease alcohol dependence	Disulfiram (Antabuse) and naltrexone (ReVia)
Panic attacks	Clonazepam (Klonopin)
Overdose with benzodiazepines	Flumazenil (Romazicon)
Hypertensive crisis from tyramine and MAOIs	Phentolamine
Atypical depression	MAOIs (eg, Phenelzine)
Narcolepsy	Modafinil (non-amphetamine stimulant)

List the *unique* toxicities of the following psychiatric drugs:

TCAs	"Three C's:" Convulsions, Cardiac arrhythmias, and Coma
Antipsychotics	Galactorrhea (from dopamine blockade)
Trazodone (Desyrel)	Priapism
Clozapine (Clozaril)	Agranulocytosis—monitor CBCs weekly; seizures
MAOIs	Hyperadrenergic/hypertensive crisis (with tyramine)
Lithium (Eskalith)	Nephrogenic DI, hypothyroidism, teratogenesis
Thioridazine (Mellaril)	Cardiac conduction abnormalities, irreversible retinal pigmentation
Chlorpromazine (Thorazine)	Corneal and lenticular deposits, jaundice, NMS
Fluphenazine (Prolixin)	Hepatotoxicity, NMS

Carbamazepine (Tegretol)	Aplastic anemia, hepatoxicity
Valproate (Depakene)	Hepatotoxicity (rare, but lethal), syndrome of inappropriate secretion of antidiuretic hormone secretion (SIADH), Stevens-Johnson syndrome, teratogenesis
Lamotrigine (Lamictal)	Stevens-Johnson syndrome, toxic epidermal necrolysis
Haloperidol (Haldol)	Arrhythmias (including torsades), NMS
Name the short-acting benzodiazepines:	"TOM is Short" Triazolam (Halcion) Oxazepam (Serax) Midazolam (Versed)
Name the intermediate-acting benzodiazepines:	"TALC" Temazepam (Restoril) Alprazolam (Xanax) Lorazepam (Ativan) Clonazepam (Klonopin)
Name the long-acting benzodiazepines:	"CD" Chlordiazepoxide (Librium) Diazepam (Valium)
Name the benzodiazepines acceptable for use in patients with hepatic dysfunction (Note: These agents are not metabolized by liver and are excreted by kidneys.)	"LOT" Lorazepam (Ativan) Oxazepam (Serax) Temazepam (Restoril) Note: chlordiazepoxide (Librium) often used for DTs if no evidence of hepatic dysfunction

MAKE THE DIAGNOSIS

20 y/o female presents with excessive anxiety about a variety of events for more than half of the days for the last 7 months.

Generalized anxiety d/o

68-y/o veteran presents with complaints of vivid flashbacks, hypervigilance, and difficulty falling asleep for the past several years; PE: patient appears very anxious.

Posttraumatic stress d/o

28-y/o male who systematically checks each lock in his house multiple times before leaving, often causing him to be over an hour late for meetings

Obsessive-compulsive d/o (OCD)

29-y/o male presents with a 9-month h/o insatiable urges to rub himself against strangers, which he has regrettably acted upon several times.

Frotteurism (sexual paraphilia)

22-y/o female college student who is 20% below her ideal body weight complains of not having any menstrual cycles and "feeling fat"

Anorexia nervosa

26-y/o female medical student for the past 9 months is convinced she has systemic lupus erythematosus (SLE) and despite numerous negative workups, she fears she will have to drop out of school.

Hypochondriasis

17-y/o female presents with complaints of "feeling fat" and h/o eating dinner alone in her bedroom; PE: normal height and weight, dental erosions, and ⊕ Russel's sign

Bulimia

24-y/o with h/o depression presents with inability to sleep, and auditory hallucinations; PE: easy distractibility and pressured speech; W/U: normal TSH and negative toxicology screen

Bipolar d/o (manic episode)

21-y/o female with no h/o trauma presents to the ER because she cannot feel or move her legs; w/u: completely within normal limits (WNL); detailed history reveals that her boyfriend of 8 years left her this morning.

Conversion d/o

43-y/o alcoholic with h/o confabulation and amnesia presents to ER after falling down; PE: nystagmus and ataxic gait; w/u: macrocytic anemia

Wernicke-Korsakoff syndrome

6-y/o presents with 8-month h/o hyperactivity, inattentiveness, and impulsivity both at school and at home; PE and w/u are essentially WNL.

ADHD

33-y/o female presents to your office distressed after turning down a lucrative job offer because of the requirement to speak in front of people.

Social phobia

9-y/o boy with 2-year h/o involuntary tics is brought to your office because he has recently been shouting obscenities.

Tourette syndrome

33-y/o female nurse presents with recent occurrences of hypoglycemia; PE: reveals multiple crossed scars on abdomen; w/u: insulin/C-peptide ratio >1.0

Factitious d/o (Munchausen syndrome)

16-y/o with h/o sudden-onset daytime sleep attacks with loss of muscle tone and audiovisual hallucinations while waking and falling asleep

Narcolepsy

19-y/o with 8-month h/o deteriorating grades and social withdrawal presents with auditory hallucinations; PE: odd thinking patterns, tangential thoughts, and flattened affect; w/u: negative toxicology screen

Schizophrenia

48-y/o female presents with recent h/o early morning waking, ↓ appetite, feelings of guilt, and loss of interest in her usual hobbies over the past 3 months; PE and labs are WNL.

Major depressive d/o

3-y/o male with h/o of poor cuddling presents with severely delayed language and social development; PE: less than normal intelligence with unusual calculating abilities, and repetitive behaviors

Autism

62-y/o man with h/o diabetes, MI, and anxiety, who recently (~1 week ago) stopped one of his medications because of insurance issues. A few days ago, he c/o nausea, vomiting, sweating, and feeling weak. Now presents w/ generalized seizure

Sedative-hypnotic withdrawal (anti-anxiety meds)

29-y/o woman with h/o multiple medical issues. Has previous negative workup for seizure disorder; chronic pain in her head, neck, back, elbows, and knees of unknown etiology; has not been able to attain orgasm for many years; and has a long history of dysphagia and "food allergies" requiring dietary restrictions

Somatization d/o

42-y/o woman presents w/a 2-year h/o the following symptoms: sweating, trembling, choking sensation, tachycardia, chest tightness, fear of losing control and dying. These symptoms develop soon after being in situations where she feels she cannot escape.

Panic attack

22-y/o woman with maladaptive coping patterns to routine stress, emotional lability, feelings of abandonment, and cutting marks on her arms and legs

Borderline personality d/o

34-y/o man with h/o schizophrenia becomes combative in the ED. He is initially managed with several doses of IM haloperidol. A few hours later he becomes agitated once again and is given high-dose ziprasidone. Soon after, he becomes delirious with unstable blood pressures. In addition, he becomes diaphoretic, febrile, and rigid, and starts to seize.

Neuroleptic malignant syndrome

11-y/o girl is having problems at school. She has trouble making friends and is awkward in social interactions. Although she has no problems with language or writing skills, she often becomes lost in the details of her school assignments and thus has difficulty completing them. When interviewed, the girl speaks in great detail about her school work, but does not make eye contact and appears uncomfortable.

Asperger syndrome

8-y/o obese boy with mental retardation, small stature, hypogonadism, compulsive eating

Prader-Willi syndrome

27-y/o woman complains of a mild chronic depressed mood that has occurred more days than not for the past 3 years. The sadness has not gone away for more than a couple of consecutive days. In addition, she denies any period of severe depression during this time.

Dysthymic d/o

CHAPTER 5

Obstetrics and Gynecology

OBSTETRICS

Complete the following formulas:

Gestational age (GA)/estimated date of confinement (EDC) =	Age of fetus from last menstrual period
No of live births/1000 people =	Birthrate
No of live births/1000 females 15-44 years old =	Fertility rate
No of neonatal deaths/1000 live births =	Neonatal mortality rate
(No of stillbirths + neonatal deaths)/1000 total births =	Perinatal mortality rate
No of infant deaths/1000 live births up to first year of life =	Infant mortality rate

Diagnosis of Pregnancy

What are typical signs and symptoms of early pregnancy?	Amenorrhea, nausea, vomiting (N/V), breast tenderness, **Chadwick's sign** (bluish discoloration and congested appearance of vagina), and **Hegar's sign** (softening of lower segment of uterus)
At what GA can fetal heart tones (FHT) be detected by Doppler?	10 weeks
At what GA can the ultrasound (US) detect a gestational sac and cardiac activity?	5 weeks and after 6 weeks, respectively

Name the three signs of fetal viability during pregnancy:	1. Fetal heart activity 2. Fetal movement detection by examiner 3. Embryo/fetus ultrasonic recognition
How early can human chorionic gonadotropin (β-hCG) be detected in urine or serum?	As early as 8-9 days after ovulation
What is the doubling time of β-hCG in early pregnancy?	2 days
When does β-hCG peak in pregnancy?	8-10 weeks GA
Name three clinical scenarios in which quantification of β-hCG is helpful:	1. Diagnosing ectopic pregnancy 2. Monitoring neoplastic trophoblastic disease 3. Screening fetal aneuploidy

Dating

What is Nägele rule?	EDC = LMP + 7 days −3 months + 1 year (based on regular 28-day cycle)
What is the most common cause of size-for-dates discrepancy?	Inaccurate dating
A definite LMP should be used to date the pregnancy if the EDC determined by a first vs second vs third TM US are within how many days of the LMP?	First trimester: 7 days Second trimester: 14 days Third trimester: 21 days

Physiologic Changes in Pregnancy

What are the physiologic changes of pregnancy in the following systems?

| Cardiovascular | ↑ heart rate (HR) and SV →↑ CO; systolic ejection murmur (SEM) is normal finding; diastolic murmur is NEVER a normal finding; ↓ BP (especially diastolic)—lowest at 24 weeks |
| Respiratory | ↑ tidal volume and minute ventilation, ↓ total lung capacity (elevation of diaphragm), ↑ total body O_2 consumption, and hyperventilation (optimizes CO_2 and O_2 transfer between mother and fetus) |

Gastrointestinal	N/V, reflux esophagitis, hemorrhoids, and cholestasis
Renal	↑ Glomerular filtration rate (GFR) 50%, ↓ BUN and Cr, urinary stasis, and asymptomatic bacteriuria in ~5%
Hematologic	↓ Hematocrit (Hct): ↑ plasma volume by 40% (due to ↑ plasma > RBC); hypercoagulable state: ↑ clotting factors (↓ protein S), ↑ venous stasis, and endothelial damage
Dermatologic	↑ estrogen → spider angiomata and palmar erythema; ↑ melanocyte stimulating hormone → hyperpigmentation of nipples, abdominal midline (linea nigra), and face (chloasma/melasma)
Endocrine	↑ hCG, human placental lactogen (hPL—insulin antagonist with diabetogenic effect), progesterone, estrogen, thyroid-binding globulin, T3 and T4 (euthyroid state), and prolactin

General Prenatal Care

What labs should be obtained at the first prenatal visit?	CBC, Rh factor, antibody screen, Pap smear, gonorrhea, and Chlamydia cultures, urinalysis (UA) and culture, rubella, syphilis, hepatitis B, HIV
Why is folate an essential part of prenatal vitamins?	Proven to ↓ risk of neural tube defects (NTD)
After 20 weeks gestation, at what rate should fundal height increase (approximately)?	1 cm per week

Teratogens

At what GA are structural abnormalities most likely to occur as a result of teratogens?	3-8 weeks since conception (organogenesis phase)

Name the teratogenic effects of the following substances:

Angiotensin-converting enzyme inhibitors (ACEi)	Renal dysgenesis → oligohydramnios, pulmonary hypoplasia, and limb contractures
Tetracycline	Discolored teeth and enamel hypoplasia
Aminoglycosides	Acoustic nerve damage → deafness
Oral hypoglycemics	Neonatal hypoglycemia
Dilantin	Fetal hydantoin syndrome: craniofacial and limb defects, mental deficiencies
Valproic acid	Spina bifida
Isotretinoin	Craniofacial (small ears), central nervous system (CNS), cardiac, and thymus defects
Indomethacin	Constriction of ductus arteriosus
Diethylstilbesterol (DES)	Clear cell vaginal cancer and cervical/uterine malformations in female offspring
Thalidomide	Limb reduction defects
Alcohol	Fetal alcohol syndrome: craniofacial defects (absent philtrum, flattened nasal bridge, microphthalmia), growth restriction, brain, cardiac, and spinal defects
Tobacco	Growth restriction
Radiation	Growth restriction, CNS defects, leukemia

ANTEPARTUM

Medical Conditions in Pregnancy

Gestational Diabetes Mellitus

What is the prevalence of gestational diabetes mellitus (GDM)?	~7% of pregnancies **Note:** most common medical complication of pregnancy
What are five risk factors for GDM?	1. >25 y/o 2. Obesity 3. ⊕ family history (FH) of diabetes mellitus (DM) 4. Previous infant >4000 g 5. Previous (h/o) polyhydramnios

How is GDM diagnosed?	Screened with glucose challenge test (50-g glucose); diagnosed with glucose tolerance test (100-g glucose)
What are three components of GDM management?	1. American Dietetic Association (ADA) diet; insulin if necessary 2. US for fetal growth assessment 3. Nonstress test (NST) starting at 30-32 weeks if requiring hypoglycemics
What is the White Classification for GDM?	A1: diet controlled A2: requiring hypoglycemics
What percentage of women with GDM will develop overt DM after their pregnancy?	>50%

Preexisting Diabetes Mellitus

How is preexisting DM managed?	Insulin, check baseline TSH, baseline ophthomology examination, baseline preeclampsia labs, monitor Hgb_{A1c}, US, and maternal serum alpha-fetoprotein (MSAFP) check at 16-20 weeks, fetal echocardiogram at 20 weeks, twice weekly NST starting at 30-32 weeks
When should elective cesarean section (CS) be considered in a patient with DM?	Fetal weight >4500 g (may consider elective delivery at 36-38 weeks with evidence of fetal lung maturity)
What are the maternal complications of DM?	Preeclampsia/eclampsia (twofold ↑ risk), hyperglycemia, retinopathy, diabetic ketoacidosis (DKA)
What are the fetal complications of DM?	Macrosomia (>4500 g), cardiac defects, caudal regression (malformations associated with poor glucose control), polyhydramnios, hypoglycemia secondary (2°) to hyperinsulinemia, intrauterine fetal death (IUFD)
What are the obstetrical complications of DM?	Preterm labor (PTL) and shoulder dystocia

Hypertension in Pregnancy

Name the hypertensive disorder (d/o) of pregnancy described below:

BP ≥140/90 before pregnancy or diagnosed before 20 weeks GA	Chronic hypertension (HTN)

BP 140/90-160/110, proteinuria 300-5000 mg/24 h, or 1-2+ on dipstick	Preeclampsia (mild)
BP >160/110, proteinuria >5000 mg/24 h, or 3-4+ on dipstick	Preeclampsia (severe)
Preeclampsia with seizures	Eclampsia
Define the HELLP syndrome:	Hemolytic anemia, Elevated (LFTs), Low Platelets
What are other signs and symptoms of severe preeclampsia/eclampsia?	Headache (HA), blurred vision, epigastric pain, hyperreflexia, and clonus
What are the risk factors for preeclampsia?	Multifetal gestation, nulliparity, ⊕ FH, maternal age <20 or >35 y/o, chronic HTN, African American, GDM, SLE
What is the management of mild preeclampsia with immature fetus?	Bed rest and monitoring of BP, weight, and serial 24° urine protein levels and preeclampsia labs (Cr, uric acid, CBC, LFTs)
What is the management of severe preeclampsia and eclampsia?	Magnesium sulfate ($MgSO_4$) until 12-24 h postpartum (PP), normalize BP, and delivery; if fetal or maternal deterioration at any gestational age → **induce labor** (delivery is the definitive treatment)

Other Medical Conditions in Pregnancy

What percentage of maternal mortalities are due to pulmonary embolism?	10% (no 1 cause of maternal death)
What is the treatment for deep venous thrombosis (DVT) or pulmonary embolism (PE) in pregnancy?	Heparin or low-molecular-weight heparin **(never warfarin!)**
What is the drug of choice for hyperthyroidism in pregnancy?	Propylthiouracil (PTU)
Why should asymptomatic bacteriuria be treated in pregnant women?	25% will develop acute, symptomatic infection if untreated
What is the most common cause of septic shock in pregnancy?	Acute pyelonephritis
What is the management of acute pyelonephritis?	*Hospitalization*, urine and blood culture, IV hydration, IV ABX, urine culture 1-2 weeks after completion of treatment/therapy (test of cure)

What is the minimum medical treatment for HIV ⊕ pregnant women?	Azidothymidine (AZT) after 14 weeks GA through labor for mom; AZT for newborn
What is the rate of vertical transmission of HIV on AZT prophylaxis?	~8% (↓ from 25% without prophylaxis)
What mode of delivery is recommended if the HIV viral load >1000 at 36 weeks GA?	Scheduled c-section
What mode of delivery is recommended in a pregnant woman with active herpes lesions during the intrapartum period?	C-section
When is universal GBS screening performed?	36 weeks GA
What anatomy must be swabbed for a complete GBS culture?	Lower vagina and rectum (through sphincter)
What is the drug of choice for GBS positive patients during the intrapartum period?	Penicillin
When GBS status is unknown, when is antibiotic treatment indicated?	GA< 36 weeks, rupture of membranes >18 hours, intrapartum temperature >38°C, h/o GBS + urine culture during current pregnancy, h/o previous infant with GBS sepsis
What is chorioamnionitis and how is it treated?	Infection of the amniotic fluid (most common cause of neonatal sepsis); broad-spectrum ABX and delivery

Obstetrical Complications

What is the differential diagnosis for bleeding in the first trimester?	Ectopic pregnancy, spontaneous abortion (SAB), postcoital bleeding, vaginal/cervical lesion, molar pregnancy, nonobstetric cause

Ectopic Pregnancy

What is the definition of an ectopic pregnancy?	Pregnancy outside uterine cavity (98% occur in the fallopian tubes)
Where do the majority of ectopic pregnancies occur	Fallopian tube (98%), most occur in ampulla

What are five risk factors for ectopic pregnancy?	1. h/o pelvic inflammatory disease (PID) or prior ectopic 2. Pelvic surgery 3. DES exposure in utero 4. Intrauterine device (IUD) usage 5. Endometriosis
What is the clinical triad of ectopic pregnancy?	1. Amenorrhea 2. Abdominal pain 3. Irregular vaginal bleeding
Name three *signs* of a ruptured ectopic pregnancy:	1. Hypotension 2. Tachycardia 3. Rebound tenderness
What is the differential diagnosis for suspected ectopic pregnancy?	Surgical abdomen, abortion, ovarian torsion, and ruptured ovarian cyst
What are four methods used to diagnose ectopic pregnancy?	1. Positive pregnancy test with empty uterus by US 2. Prolonged hCG doubling 3. Progesterone <25 ng/mL 4. Surgical abdomen
What medication can be offered for a stable, unruptured ectopic pregnancy <3.5 cm and <6 weeks GA?	Methotrexate
What is the definitive treatment for most other ectopic pregnancies?	Laparoscopic surgery

Abortion

Define spontaneous abortion (SAB) or miscarriage:	Loss of pregnancy before 20 weeks GA or delivery of fetus <500 g
Name the type of abortion described below (all <20 weeks GA) and appropriate treatment:	
Intrauterine bleeding *without* dilation of cervix and no expulsion of products of conception (POC)	Threatened **Tx:** after documenting a live fetus, pelvic rest
Intrauterine bleeding *with* dilation of cervix and no expulsion of POC	Inevitable **Tx:** surgical evacuation of uterine contents
Partial expulsion of POC	Incomplete **Tx:** possible hospitalization, possible hemodynamic resuscitation, and curettage

Complete expulsion of POC	Complete
	Tx: none
Death of embryo/fetus with retention of POC	Missed
	Tx: surgical evacuation of uterine contents if there is no spontaneous resolution
≥2 consecutive or three total SABs	Recurrent
	Tx: based on type of abortion

What is the most common cause of a first trimester fetal death?	Chromosomal abnormality
What are signs/symptoms of SAB?	Vaginal bleeding, cramping, abdominal pain, decreased signs or symptoms of pregnancy
What is the most common method of surgical evacuation of uterine contents in the first and second trimesters?	First trimester: dilation and curettage (D&C) Second trimester: dilation and evacuation

Antepartum and Intrapartum Hemorrhage

Half of all third trimester bleeding is caused by what two conditions?	1. Placental abruption 2. Placenta previa
What is a rare but important cause of third trimester bleeding involving the fetus?	Vasa previa
Define placental abruption	Premature separation of normally implanted placenta
Name eight risk factors for placental abruption:	1. HTN 2. ↑ maternal age 3. Multiparity 4. African American 5. Preterm premature rupture of membranes (PPROM) 6. Smoking tobacco 7. Cocaine use 8. Trauma
What are the signs and symptoms of placental abruption?	*Painful* bleeding, contractions, and fetal distress/death
How is placental abruption diagnosed?	Clinically; there is a high suspicion if placenta previa is ruled out by US

How is placental abruption managed?	Hemodynamic support, RhoGAM if appropriate, hospitalization; bed rest if preterm; induction of mature fetus or C-section if unstable fetus or mother
What are four complications of placental abruption?	1. Hypovolemic shock 2. Disseminated intravascular coagulation (DIC) 3. Preterm delivery 4. Fetal death
Define placenta previa:	Implantation of placenta over cervical os (complete, partial, or marginal)
Name four risk factors for placenta previa:	1. h/o C-section 2. Age >35 years 3. Multiparity 4. Smoking
What is the most common sign of placenta previa?	*Painless* bleeding
How is placenta previa diagnosed?	Ultrasound
How is placenta previa managed?	Hemodynamic support, RhoGAM if appropriate, expectant management; delivery by CS if fetus is mature or if patient is unstable
Name four complications of placenta previa:	1. Hypovolemic shock 2. Preterm delivery 3. ↑ fetal anomalies (2×) 4. Placenta accreta
Define *placenta accreta* and its variants, *increta* and *percreta*:	*Accreta*: placenta abnormally **A**ttaches to myometrium *Increta*: **I**nvades myometrium *Percreta*: **P**enetrates through myometrium to serosa
What are four risk factors for placenta accreta?	1. Placenta previa 2. h/o c-section 3. h/o curettage 4. Gravida six or more
What are the signs and symptoms of placenta accreta?	Antepartum bleeding (if associated with placenta previa, otherwise asymptomatic)
How is placenta accreta diagnosed?	US or MRI (false positive can occur with both)

How is placenta accreta managed?	Uterine packing to stop PP bleeding or hysterectomy
Define vasa previa:	Fetal vessels passing over the internal cervical os → cord compression and possibly, rupture
What is the incidence of fetal mortality if the fetal vessel ruptures?	>50%
What is a major risk factor for vasa previa?	Velamentous cord insertion with multiple gestation
What fetal tracing is associated with ruptured fetal vessel?	Sinusoidal wave (indicating fetal anemia)
What is the treatment for vasa previa?	Emergent c-section
What is a rare but devastating cause of bleeding associated with abdominal pain during labor?	Uterine rupture
What are four risk factors for uterine rupture?	1. Prior c-section 2. Trauma 3. Overdistented uterus 4. Abnormal placentation

Preterm Labor

What is preterm labor (PTL)?	Labor before 37 weeks GA
What are eight risk factors for PTL?	1. Preterm rupture of membranes 2. h/o PTL 3. Infection 4. Multiple gestation 5. Uterine or fetal anomaly 6. Preeclampsia 7. Low socioeconomic status 8. Smoking tobacco
What are the clinical predictors of PTL?	Persistent uterine contractions, fetal fibronectin (if negative, can help rule out PTL), ongoing cervical dilation >3 cm or effacement >80%, vaginal bleeding, and ruptured membranes
What are the positive and negative predictive values (PPV and NPV) for delivery within 14 days for fetal fibronectin?	PPV: 16%; NPV: 99%

How is PTL managed?	Hydration, empiric ABX if GBS unknown, tocolysis, and steroids if fetus 24-34 weeks GA or negative fetal lung maturity test between 34 and 37 weeks GA
Name four tocolytic agents:	1. $MgSO_4$ 2. Nifedipine 3. Indomethacin 4. Terbutaline
Name three serious toxicities of $MgSO_4$:	1. Loss of reflexes 2. Respiratory depression 3. Cardiac arrest
What is the treatment for Mg toxicity?	Calcium gluconate

What are common side effects of:

Nifedipine	Headache
Indocin	Oligohydramnios
Terbutaline	Hypoglycemia and tachycardia

Premature Rupture of Membranes

Define premature rupture of membranes (PROM):	Spontaneous rupture of membranes before onset of labor; if occurring preterm → PPROM
How is PROM diagnosed?	"Gush of fluid" per vagina, sterile speculum examination (avoid digital examination) to visualize dilation/ effacement; positive pool, nitrazine (alkaline blue), or ferning test
How is PROM managed?	If there are signs of chorioamnionitis (fever, ↑ WBC, maternal/fetal tachycardia, uterine tenderness) treat with antibiotics and delivery; induction of labor within 24 h of PROM if failure to progress
How is PPROM managed?	Hospitalization, bedrest, antibiotics (to prevent infection and to delay labor), +/− steroids
What is prolonged rupture of membranes?	Rupture of membranes lasting >18 h before delivery

| What is the major fetal complication associated with PPROM at ≤26 weeks GA? | Pulmonary hypoplasia |

Amniotic Fluid Abnormalities

What term is used to describe an amniotic fluid index (AFI) <5?	Oligohydramnios
What are the two basic mechanisms of oligohydramnios?	1. ↓ fetal urine output 2. Chronic leak through membranes
What conditions are associated with oligohydramnios?	Congenital abnormalities, ruptured membranes, uteroplacental insufficiency, HTN, DM, ACEi, or NSAID usage, postterm pregnancy, and twin-twin transfusion syndrome
What term is used to describe AFI >25?	Polyhydramnios
What are the three basic mechanisms of polyhydramnios?	1. ↑ fetal urine output 2. ↓ fetal swallowing 3. Transudation of fluid from exposed meninges (as in spina bifida)
What conditions are associated with polyhydramnios?	NTD, alimentary canal defect, hydrops, DM, and twin-twin transfusion syndrome

Rh Incompatibility

If the mother is Rh−Rh− and the father is Rh+Rh+, what percentage of their offspring will be Rh+?	100%
If the mother is Rh−Rh− and the father is Rh+Rh−, what percentage of their offspring will be Rh+?	50%
If a woman is Rh−Rh−, by what mechanism can she become anti-D (IgG) positive?	Previous pregnancy, blood transfusion, trauma in current pregnancy
What is the effect of anti-D on an Rh+ fetus?	Anti-D can cross the placenta and cause hemolysis of fetal RBCs.
Name the fetal condition characterized by severe hemolytic anemia resulting in a hyperdynamic state, heart failure, diffuse edema, ascites, and pericardial effusion:	Erythroblastosis fetalis

Which patients should receive RhoGAM and why?	Rh–/Ab– women at risk for being pregnant with Rh+ fetus
At what gestational age should pregnant women receive RhoGAM even without a history of bleeding?	28 weeks

Multiple Gestation

What is the term given to fetal twins resulting from fertilization of two ova?	Dizygotic (always two amnion and two chorion)
What is the term given to twins resulting from one fertilized ovum that divides into two?	Monozygotic twins
Ethnicity (especially African descent), ↑ age, ↑ parity, and FH are contributing factors to ↑ monozygotic or dizygotic twinning?	Dizygotic

For the following types of monozygotic twins, how many days after fertilization did the ovum likely divide?

Two chorion, two amnion (DiDi), two placenta	2-3 days (before trophoblastic differentiation)
One chorion, two amnion (MoDi), one placenta	3-8 days
One chorion, one amnion (MoMo), one placenta	8-13 days
Conjoined twins	13-15 days (after formation of embryonic disk)

What signs or symptoms should raise the suspicion of a multiple gestation pregnancy?	Uterus larger than dates, excess maternal weight gain, hydramnios or unexplained maternal anemia, auscultation of more than one fetal heart, h/o ovulation induction or in vitro fertilization (IVF); confirmation by US
What syndrome in monochorionic twins occurs when the arterial circulation of one twin is in communication with the venous circulation of the other?	Twin-to-twin transfusion syndrome

What are sonographic findings of dichorionic, diamnionic twins?	Two placentas, twin peak sign, and thick inter-twin membrane
Describe the differences between the donor and recipient twin in twin-to-twin transfusion syndrome:	**Donor:** anemia, growth restriction, and oligohydramnios **Recipient:** polycythemia, hypervolemic, cardiomegaly, and congestive heart failure (CHF)
How are twins delivered?	If first twin is vertex and second twin is not significantly larger, then trial of labor (TOL); otherwise CS
What is the most common cause of postterm pregnancy?	Inaccurate dating
What two congenital abnormalities are associated with postterm pregnancy?	Anencephaly and adrenal hypoplasia

Fetal Diagnostic Testing and Monitoring

What are the indications for prenatal genetic analysis of a fetus?	Advanced maternal age (AMA), ⊕ FH or previous child with chromosomal abnormality, fetal abnormality on US, abnormal serum marker screening, and unexplained intrauterine growth retardation (IUGR)
What screening tests are available for prenatal diagnosis of genetic abnormalities?	Sequential screen (first trimester nuchal translucency with blood draw plus second trimester blood draw) and quadruple screen (second trimester blood draw)
At what gestational age do you perform a nuchal translucency?	10-14 weeks
What four parameters are tested in a quad screen?	1. MSAFP 2. Estriol 3. hCG 4. Inhibin A
Name five causes of elevated MSAFP:	1. *NTD* 2. Inaccurate dating 3. Multiple gestation 4. Fetal abdominal wall defect 5. Fetal death

What three tests are available for checking a fetal karyotype?	1. Amniocentesis 2. Chorionic villus sampling (CVS) 3. Percutaneous umbilical blood sampling (PUBS)
At what gestational age is an amniocentesis performed and what is the incidence of complications?	16-21 weeks GA; 1/200-1/300
At what gestational age is CVS performed and what is the incidence of complications?	9-11 weeks GA; 0.5%-1%
What is the advantage of CVS over amniocentesis?	Offers prenatal genetic diagnosis in the first trimester and allows earlier and safer pregnancy termination if desired
What is a rare fetal complication of CVS?	Limb reduction defects
In addition to karyotype, what information does a cordocentesis reveal?	Fetal hematocrit, platelet count, and fetal blood type
What two tests are commonly used to assess fetal lung maturity?	1. Lecithin/sphingomyelin ratio >2 2. Presence of phosphatidylglycerol in amniotic fluid **Note:** both obtained by amniocentesis
What constitutes a reactive NST?	≥2 accelerations (increased HR), each ≥15 bpm above the baseline for ≥15 s, all within 20 min
What are the five parameters of a biophysical profile (BPP)?	"Test the Baby, **MAN!**" 1. **T**one (extension/flexion of limb) 2. **B**reathing 3. Goss **M**ovement 4. **A**FI 5. **N**ST
When is a BPP performed?	When the NST is non-reactive or equivocal
What is a normal BPP score?	8-10

INTRAPARTUM

Normal Labor and delivery

Triage

What is the term for irregular contractions not associated with cervical dilation or effacement?	Braxton Hicks contractions or false labor
What is the term for regular uterine contractions that cause progressive cervical dilation and/or effacement?	Labor
Name three ways to confirm rupture of membranes on vaginal examination:	1. Positive pooling (low sensitivity) 2. Ferning test 3. Nitrazine test (turns blue due to increased pH)
Do blood, semen, and vaginitis cause a false–positive- or a false-negative nitrazine test?	False positive
Name five parameters evaluated on cervical examination to produce a Bishop's score:	1. Dilation 2. Effacement 3. Station 4. Consistency 5. Position
What is the most common fetal presentation?	Vertex, occiput anterior

Progression of Labor

What are the cardinal movements of labor?	Engagement, descent, flexion, internal rotation, extension, external rotation (restitution), and expulsion
Define the following stages of labor:	
First stage	Onset of labor → full cervical dilation (10 cm)
First stage: latent phase	Onset of labor → ~4 cm cervical dilation
First stage: active phase	~4 cm → 10 cm (rapid dilation)
Second stage	Complete cervical dilation → delivery of infant
Third stage	Delivery of infant → delivery of placenta (should be <30 min)

What are the three signs of placental separation?	1. Rising and firming of uterus 2. Gush of blood 3. Umbilical cord lengthening

Identify the degree of laceration described below:

Involving the skin or mucosa	First degree
Involving the fascia and muscles of perineal body	Second degree
Involving the anal sphincter	Third degree
Involving the anal mucosa (exposing lumen of rectum)	Fourth degree

Intrapartum Fetal Assessment

What is the normal range of a fetal HR (FHR)?	120-160 bpm
What is the differential diagnosis for fetal bradycardia?	Fetal distress, local anesthetics, and congenital heart block (seen with maternal SLE)
What is the differential diagnosis for fetal tachycardia?	Fetal infection or arrhythmia; maternal fever, anxiety or thyrotoxicosis; terbutaline; fetal movement and stimulation
What is the definition of a reactive FHR tracing?	≥ 2 accelerations ($\uparrow$ in HR), each ≥ 15 bpm above the baseline for ≥ 15 s, all within 20 min

Identify the following three types of decelerations and name their etiologies:

Symmetric deceleration that begins and ends at around the same time as contractions; looks like "mirror image" of contraction	Early deceleration; due to **head compression** stimulating vagus nerve
Most common; sharp drop and return to baseline, often preceded and followed by an acceleration (*shoulders*) and occurring at any time	Variable deceleration; due to **cord compression**
Begins at the peak of a contraction and slowly returns to the baseline after the end of a contraction	Late deceleration; due to **uteroplacental insufficiency**

Which type of deceleration is most worrisome, requiring intervention if it becomes repetitive?	Late deceleration
Which type of deceleration is normal and requires no intervention?	Early deceleration
Which type of deceleration is abnormal and requires intervention depending on its severity?	Variable deceleration
Name an alternative test to fetal scalp blood sampling:	Scalp stimulation (digital stroking of fetal scalp that evokes an acceleration suggests normal scalp pH)

Abnormal Labor and Delivery

What is the term for initiating labor in a nonlaboring patient?	Induction
What are the most common indications for labor induction?	**Maternal:** Preeclampsia and DM **Fetal:** chorioamnionitis, IUGR, postterm, and hydrops
Name three methods used to promote cervical maturation (or ripening), which would improve induction results:	1. Prostaglandin gel/insert 2. Laminaria 3. Intrauterine Foley balloon
Name two common methods used to induce labor:	1. Pitocin (oxytocin) 2. Amniotomy
Name two complications associated with pitocin:	1. Uterine hyperstimulation (stop pitocin, left lateral position, O_2) 2. Water intoxication (prevent with strict I/O management)
What term is used to describe strengthening contractions in a laboring patient?	Augmentation
Name two methods used to augment labor:	1. Pitocin 2. Amniotomy
What must be confirmed prior to performing amniotomy	Engagement of fetal head into maternal pelvis
What term is used to describe difficult labor?	Dystocia

What are the "three P's" associated with dystocia?	Abnormalities of: 1. **Power:** uterine contractility and maternal expulsive effort (poor) 2. **Passenger:** fetus (malpresentation, breech presentation, shoulder impaction, hydrocephalus) 3. **Passage:** pelvis (android and platypelloid pelvic types, uterine fibroid)
Name the following types of breeches (buttock presentation):	
Flexed hips and extended feet → feet are near fetal head	Frank (most common)
Flexed hips and one or two flexed knees → at least 1 foot near breech	Complete
One or two hips extended → at least 1 foot below breech	Footling (least common)
How is full-term, laboring, and breech usually managed?	c-section
What two other methods are used to manage breech presentation?	1. External cephalic version 2. Trial of vaginal delivery
Define shoulder dystocia:	Impaction of shoulder behind pubic symphysis after delivered head
What are the risk factors for shoulder dystocia?	Macrosomia, GDM, maternal obesity, and postterm delivery
What are the fetal complications of shoulder dystocia?	Fracture of humerus/clavicle, brachial plexus injury (Erb's palsy), hypoxia, and death
Name the following maneuvers that can help displace the shoulder impaction:	
Pressure on maternal abdomen behind pubic symphysis	Suprapubic pressure
Sharp flexion of maternal hips	McRoberts maneuver
Pressure on posterior shoulder, rotating it in corkscrew fashion	Woods corkscrew maneuver
Pressure on accessible shoulder, pushing it toward anterior chest and decreasing shoulder-shoulder diameter	Rubin maneuver

Sweep posterior shoulder across chest, delivering arm, and rotate shoulder girdle to oblique diameter of pelvis	Delivery of posterior shoulder
Fracture of clavicle	Fracture of clavicle (last resort)
Replace infant's head back in pelvis and perform CS	Zavanelli maneuver (last resort)

What are the four most common indications for CS?	1. Prior CS 2. Labor dystocia 3. Fetal distress 4. Breech presentation
Women with what kind of prior uterine incision are candidates for vaginal birth after cesarean (VBAC) trial of labor (TOL)?	Low transverse, low vertical
What is the major complication associated with VBAC?	Uterine rupture

POSTPARTUM

Complications

What is the definition of postpartum (PP) hemorrhage?	Loss of ≥500 cc blood after completion of third stage of labor
What are the three most common causes of PP hemorrhage?	1. Uterine atony 2. Retained placenta 3. Cervical/vaginal laceration
What are the risk factors for uterine atony?	Uterine overdistension (multiple gestation, hydramnios, macrosomia), multiparity, general anesthesia, and h/o PP hemorrhage
Describe the management of PP hemorrhage:	Uterine massage → oxytocin, methergine, or prostaglandin → explore uterus for retained placenta and explore cervix and vagina for lacerations → surgical intervention
What are the surgical interventions for PP hemorrhage?	Postpartum D&C, uterine artery embolization, and hysterectomy

What are three symptoms of PP endometritis?	1. Fever ≥38°C (100.4°F) within 36 h of delivery 2. Uterine tenderness 3. Malodorous lochi
What are six risk factors for PP endometritis?	1. Delivery by CS 2. Low socioeconomic status 3. Young age 4. Prolonged ruptured membranes 5. Bacterial colonization of lower genital tract 6. Steroids
What is the treatment for PP endometritis?	Broad-spectrum ABX until afebrile for 24 h
What kind of contraception is appropriate when a mother is breastfeeding?	Progestin-only pills, Depo-Provera Mirena or Paraguard IUD, and Implanon
Name the following PP psychologic reactions:	
Mild to suicidal depression that begins at ~4 weeks PP and can last up to 1 year PP	PP depression (may affect up to 20% of PP mothers)
Transient symptoms of depression that usually resolve by PP day 10	Maternity/PP blues (may affect up to 70% of PP mothers)
What clinical assessment tool is used to help diagnose postpartum depression?	Edinburgh depression scale

GYNECOLOGY

Benign Gynecology

Menstruation

Describe the endocrine changes that occur during each of the following phases of menstruation:	
Follicular phase (proliferative, days 1-14)	1. Follicle-stimulating hormone (FSH) → follicular development 2. Estrogen → endometrial proliferation and then FSH suppression 3. Progesterone low

Ovulation (day 15)	Estrogen-induced luteinizing hormone (LH) surge → ovulation
Luteal phase (secretory, days 15-28)	1. Corpus luteum secrete progesterone → endometrium maturation 2. ↓ LH and FSH 3. Corpus luteum regress →↓ progesterone and estrogen
What condition is characterized by painful cramping in the lower abdomen, with sweating, N/V, and HA—all occurring just before or during menses?	Dysmenorrhea
What is the treatment for primary dysmenorrhea?	NSAIDs, oral contraceptive pills (OCP)
What is the treatment for secondary dysmenorrhea?	Treat underlying disease (endometriosis, PID, ovarian cyst, fibroids)
What is the term for somatic and psychologic symptoms that occur in the second half of the menstrual cycle, interfere with work and personal relationships, and are followed by symptom-free periods?	Premenstrual dysphoric disorder (PMDD)
Name some characteristic physical symptoms of PMDD:	Bloating, breast pain, skin disorders, HA, pelvic pain, N/V, edema, and cravings
Name some characteristic psychologic symptoms of PMDD:	Irritability, aggression, tension, anxiety, sadness, mood lability, and depression
Name six treatment options for the symptoms of PMDD:	1. Diet and exercise 2. Selective serotonin reuptake inhibitor (SSRI) 3. Diuretic for edema 4. OCPs 5. Support bra for breast pain 6. Reassurance

Abnormal Uterine Bleeding

Name the term used to describe the following types of abnormal uterine bleeding:	
Heavy (>80 cc) or prolonged (>7 days) occurring at normal intervals	Menorrhagia

Irregular menstrual bleeding	Metrorrhagia
Frequent periods	Polymenorrhea
Menses >35 days apart	Oligomenorrhea
Absence of menstrual bleeding	Amenorrhea (pregnancy is most common cause)

What is the workup for abnormal uterine bleeding?	1. Exclude pregnancy 2. Rule out structural etiology 3. Consider dysfunctional uterine bleeding, such as anovulatory source
What is the differential diagnosis for menorrhagia and metrorrhagia?	"LACCE" Leiomyoma Adenomyosis Cervical cancer Coagulopathy Endometrial hyperplasia, or endometriosis, polyps, cancer

Contraception/Sterilization

What is the general mechanism of action (MOA) of OCP?	Ovulation suppression **Estrogen:** inhibits FSH → prevents selection and maturation of dominant follicle **Progestin:** inhibits LH → prevents ovulation
What are three other MOAs of both combination and progestin-only formulations?	1. Thicken cervical mucus 2. ↓ fallopian tube motility 3. Cause endometrial atrophy
What are the *advantages* of OCPs?	<1% failure rate with perfect use, usually ↓ cramping, protect against ovarian and endometrial cancer, ↓ PID and ectopic pregnancies, ↓ bone loss, and cause lighter menstrual flow
What are the *disadvantages* of OCPs?	Daily pill; no protection against STDs; **side effects:** ↑ risk of irregular bleeding, nausea, irritability, amenorrhea, and breast tenderness; thrombosis; myocardial infarction (MI); cerebrovascular accident (CVA); and gallstones
What are the *contraindications* to OCPs?	Pregnancy, h/o thromboembolic d/o or stroke, chronic liver disease, undiagnosed uterine bleeding, breast cancer/carcinoma (CA), endometrial CA, smoking in women >35 y/o

How many hours after intercourse must OCPs be taken to act as emergency contraception?	Within 72 h (repeat in 12 h)
What are the *advantages* of progestin-only pills (*mini-pills*)?	Ideal for nursing mothers and women who cannot take estrogen for medical reasons
What are the *disadvantages* of progestin-only pills?	Higher failure rate (3%-6%), strict compliance necessary (must take pill same time everyday)
What are other methods of combined estrogen and progesterone contraceptives besides OCPs?	Vaginal contraceptive ring and the transdermal contraceptive patch
What is the name of the single-rod contraceptive implant?	Implanon
What slow-releasing, IM injection of progesterone is given every 3 months for contraception?	Depo-Provera
What are the side effects of Depo-Provera?	Irregular bleeding, conception delayed 9 months following last injection, HA, and weight gain
What is the mechanism of action (MOA) of the levonorgestrel IUD?	Levonorgestrel causes thickened cervical mucous making sperm unable to come in contact with the ovum.
What is MOA of the copper IUD?	Copper works as a functional spermacide, inhibiting sperm motility and acrosomal enzyme activation.
What are the side effects of the levonorgestrel IUD?	Irregular bleeding during the first 3-6 months, ovarian cysts, acne, mood alteration
What are the side effects of the copper IUD?	Increased menstrual bleeding and cramping
What are four methods of permanent sterilization?	1. Tubal ligation 2. Hysteroscopic sterilization (Essure) 3. Hysterectomy (not done for sole purpose of permanent sterilization) 4. Vasectomy for men

Menopause

What is the definition of menopause?	No menses for >1 year
What is the mean age of menopause in the United States?	51 years
What are the signs and symptoms of perimenopause and menopause?	Hot flashes, irritability, insomnia, depression, memory loss, dyspareunia, urinary urgency, vaginal atrophy, and ↓ bone mass
How is menopause diagnosed?	Based on history, ↑ FSH
Name the three indications for hormone replacement therapy (HRT):	1. Treatment of vasomotor symptoms 2. Prevention of osteoporosis (raloxifene a better choice) 3. Relief of genitourinary symptoms (topical estrogens preferred)
What are five *contraindications* to HRT?	1. Uterine bleeding of unknown origin 2. Liver disease 3. h/o DVT or PE 4. h/o breast CA 5. h/o endometrial CA
Based on the Women's Health Initiative, HRT is no longer indicated to prevent what disease?	Coronary heart disease

Infections

What age group has the highest incidence of PID in the United States?	15-25 years
Aside from age what are the other risk factors for PID?	Multiple sexual partners, new sexual partner, unprotected intercourse, h/o STD, and h/o invasive gynecologic procedures
Name two organisms that cause the majority of PID cases:	1. *Neisseria gonorrhoeae* 2. *Chlamydia trachomatis* Note: *Escherichia coli* and *Bacteroides* cause most of the remainder of cases.
What signs are likely to be found on PE in PID?	Abdominal tenderness, adnexal tenderness, elevated temperature, and cervical motion tenderness (*chandelier sign*)

What is the differential diagnosis for *acute* pelvic pain?	**"A ROPE"** **A**ppendicitis **R**uptured ovarian cyst **O**varian torsion/abscess **P**ID **E**ctopic pregnancy
What are the criteria for hospitalization in PID?	Pregnancy, peritonitis, N/V, or abscess (tuboovarian or pelvic)
What is the treatment of PID?	Broad-spectrum cephalosporin and doxycycline (*Chlamydia* coverage)
What condition presents with right upper quadrant (RUQ) pain, fever, N/V, and a significant h/o PID?	Fitz-Hugh-Curtis syndrome
Name the cause of vaginitis and appropriate treatment in each of the following clinical scenarios:	
Positive whiff test and clue cells on wet prep	Bacterial vaginosis **Tx:** metronidazole
Pruritis and erythema, white discharge, pseudohyphae in 10% KOH	*Candida* → azole **Tx:** antifungals
Pruritis, frothy discharge, motile and flagellated organisms on wet prep, "strawberry cervix"	*Trichomonas* → metronidazole (must treat partner) **Tx:** metronidazole
What is the treatment for a Bartholin gland abscess?	Incision and drainage (I&D), Word catheter for drainage, warm sitz baths; marsupialization for refractory disease

Endometriosis/Adenomyosis

What disorder is characterized by the growth of functional endometrial glands and stroma outside of the uterus?	Endometriosis
What is the typical parity and age of a patient with endometriosis?	Nulliparous females in twenties and thirties
Where is endometriosis most commonly found?	Uterosacral ligaments, cul-de-sac, ovaries, fallopian tubes, cervix, and colon (rarely in lungs, bladder, kidney, spine, arms, and legs)

Name two classic symptoms of endometriosis:	1. Cyclic pelvic pain (lesions stimulated by estrogen) 2. Dyspareunia
Name three classic signs of endometriosis:	1. Fixed retroverted uterus (by adhesions) 2. Nodularity of uterosacral ligaments and cul-de-sac 3. Tender ovarian masses
What is the differential diagnosis for *chronic* pelvic pain?	Irritable bowel syndrome, interstitial cystitis, fibromyalgia, degenerating myomas, primary dysmenorrhea, depression, and prior psychiatric abuse
How is the diagnosis of endometriosis confirmed?	Laparoscopic visualization and biopsy
What is the term for the classic lesion filled with dark, old blood and found on the ovary in patients with endometriitis?	Chocolate cyst (endometrioma)
What is the term for old, end-stage endometriotic lesions?	Black or powder burn
What are three medical treatment options for endometriosis?	1. Hormonal contraception 2. Gonadotropin-releasing hormone (GnRH) agonist (Lupron) 3. Androgen agonist (Danazol)
What are the surgical procedures for the treatment of endometriosis?	Lysis of adhesions and excision of endometriomas for those who want to preserve fertility; total hysterectomy and bilateral salpingo-oophorectomy (TAHBSO) for severe disease
What term describes the condition in which endometrial tissue is found within the myometrium?	Adenomyosis
Adenomyosis peaks in which decades?	Forties and fifties (commonly in multiparous females)
What is the triad of symptoms in adenomyosis?	1. Dysmenorrhea (noncyclic) 2. Menorrhagia 3. Enlarged uterus
What is the differential diagnosis of adenomyosis?	Myomas, dysfunctional uterine bleeding, and pregnancy with bleeding

What is the definitive method of diagnosis and ultimate treatment of adenomyosis?	Hysterectomy

Leiomyoma/Leiomyosarcoma

What is the most common pelvic tumor?	Leiomyoma (myoma/fibroid) = benign neoplasm of smooth muscle
What is the prevalence of leiomyomas in white and black women?	Found in 25% of white women and 50% of black women (usually of reproductive age)
Name five types of degenerations a leiomyoma may undergo once it outgrows its blood supply:	1. Hyaline 2. Myxomatous 3. Calcific 4. Red (painful hemorrhage often with pregnancy) 5. Cystic
What symptoms are associated with leiomyoma?	Abnormal uterine bleeding and pelvic pressure (majority, however, are asymptomatic)
How are leiomyomas diagnosed?	Usually by bimanual pelvic examination; imaging: US, abdominal x-ray (concentric calcifications), CT and MRI (rarely necessary)
What are the surgical options for unremitting, symptomatic leiomyomas?	Myomectomy and uterine artery emoblization for patients who wish to preserve fertility, otherwise hysterectomy

Ovarian Cyst

What is the most common type of functional ovarian cyst?	Follicular cyst (usually asymptomatic)
What type of ovarian cyst develops bilaterally in response to elevated hCG levels?	Theca lutein cyst
How are ovarian cysts diagnosed?	Pelvic examination and US
What is the differential diagnosis for an adnexal mass?	Ovarian cyst, ectopic pregnancy, ovarian torsion, tuboovarian abscess (TOA), endometrioma, fibroid, and ovarian neoplasm

Pelvic Mass

What is the most likely diagnosis
for a pelvic mass associated with the
following findings?

Painless, heavy uterine bleeding   Leiomyoma

Amenorrhea   Pregnancy

Dysmenorrhea   Endometriosis, adenomyosis, ectopic
                                          pregnancy, corpus luteum with
                                          endometrioma

Postmenopausal   Ovarian cancer

Significant h/o PID   TOA

GYNECOLOGY ONCOLOGY

Vulvar Dysplasia and Cancer

What are the signs and symptoms   Pruritis, raised white lesion, ulceration,
of vulvar cancer (CA)?   exophytic mass, and bleeding (most are
                                          asymptomatic)

How is vulvar cancer diagnosed?   Biopsy any suspicious lesion

What is the most common histologic   Squamous cell carcinoma
type of vulvar cancer?

Cervical Dysplasia and Cancer

What are the risk factors for cervical   Human papillomavirus (HPV) infection
dysplasia and cervical cancer?   (especially types 16, 18, 31, 33), early
                                          intercourse, multiple sex partners, low
                                          socioeconomic status, cigarette smoking,
                                          and HIV

What is the most important screening   Pap smear
tool for cervical dysplasia and cancer?

What are the guidelines for initiating   Start annual Pap smear on every woman
routine Pap smears?   >21 y/o or within 3 years of onset of
                                          sexual activity

What are the two major types of   1. Squamous cell carcinoma (90%)
cervical cancers?   2. Adenocarcinoma (including clear cell
                                             carcinoma from DES exposure)

| What are five symptoms of cervical cancer? | 1. Postcoital bleeding
2. Irregular bleeding
3. Lower extremity edema
4. Renal failure
5. Pelvic pain/pressure |

| Which cancer is the only gynecologic cancer that is staged clinically and not surgically? | Cervical cancer |

Describe the general anatomic spread of cervical cancer in each of the following stages:

Stage I	Confined to cervix
Stage II	Extends beyond cervix but not to pelvic wall, involves upper two-thirds of vagina
Stage III	Extends to pelvic wall, involves lower one-third of vagina and/or causes hydronephrosis or nonfunctioning kidney
Stage IV	Extends beyond pelvis, involves bladder or colon mucosa

| What are treatment options for cervical cancer? | Conization, trachelectomy, radical hysterectomy, primary chemoradiation and ajuvant chemoradiation. Tx options depend on stage and patient's desire to preserve fertility. |

Endometrial Hyperplasia and Cancer

| What are six major risk factors for endometrial hyperplasia and endometrial cancer? | Unopposed estrogen exposure:
1. Obesity
2. Nulliparity
3. Late menopause >55 years
4. Chronic anovulation
5. Polycystic ovarian syndrome (PCOS)
6. Tamoxifen |

| What is the typical presentation of endometrial hyperplasia? | Abnormal uterine bleeding or oligomenorrhea |

| How is endometrial hyperplasia diagnosed? | Endometrial biopsy or D&C |

| What is the treatment for endometrial hyperplasia? | Progestin therapy for simple, complex, and atypical simple hyperplasia; TAHBSO for atypical complex hyperplasia |

What is the most common gynecologic cancer in the United States?	Endometrial cancer
What is the most common symptom of endometrial cancer?	Postmenopausal bleeding (>90%)
What is the differential diagnosis for postmenopausal bleeding?	Endometrial hyperplasia or cancer, uterine/cervical polyp, exogenous estrogens, cervical CA, and atrophic vaginitis (if older patient, must rule out malignancy)
How is endometrial cancer diagnosed?	Endometrial biopsy
What percentage of women with postmenopausal bleeding will have endometrial cancer?	10%
What four surgical procedures are involved in the staging of endometrial cancer?	1. Explanatory laparotomy 2. TAHBSO 3. Pelvic washing (cytology) 4. Pelvic and aortic lymph node dissection

Ovarian Cancer

Which gynecologic cancer has the highest mortality rate?	Ovarian cancer (usually diagnosed at Stage III or IV)
What are the three basic histologic types of ovarian cancers?	1. Epithelial 2. Germ cell 3. Sex cord-stromal

Epithelial

Epithelial ovarian cancer accounts for what percentage of ovarian malignancies?	90%
What are the risk factors for ovarian cancer?	Advanced age, Caucasian race, nulliparity, and FH of breast colon or ovarian cancer
What are the protective factors for ovarian cancer?	Breastfeeding, OCP, tubal ligation, hysterectomy, and multiparity
What are the early and late stage signs of ovarian cancer?	**Early:** asymptomatic **Late:** pelvic mass, fluid wave, bowel obstruction

What are the three goals of surgery in epithelial ovarian cancer?	1. Establish diagnosis 2. Stage (extent of disease) 3. Debulk all visible disease if advanced cancer (include TAHBSO and nodes)
Name two adjuvant chemotherapies for epithelial ovarian cancer:	1. Carboplatin 2. Paclitaxel

Nonepithelial

What two histologic types comprise the nonepithelial tumors?	1. Germ cell tumors (GCT) 2. Sex cord-stromal tumors
What percent of GCTs are benign?	95%
In what age group are GCTs usually diagnosed?	Teens and twenties
GCTs arise from what kind of cells?	Totipotential germ cells
What are the signs and symptoms of GCTs?	May grow rapidly → pain from distension, torsion, or hemorrhage; adnexal mass, ascites, and pleural effusion
What ethnicities are at greater risk for development of GCTs?	Asians/African Americans

Describe the general anatomic spread of ovarian cancer in each of the following stages:

Stage I	Limited to ovaries
Stage II	Extension from ovaries to pelvis
Stage III	Extension to abdominal cavity
Stage IV	Distant metastatic disease

Name the type of GCTs characterized by each of the following statements:

Most common malignant GCT; may be bilateral; ↑ LDH; excellent prognosis	Dysgerminoma
Yolk sac tumor; Schiller-Duval bodies; ↑ alpha-fetoprotein (AFP); poor prognosis	Endodermal sinus tumor

Comprise 30% of all ovarian neoplasms; benign cystic teratoma; struma ovarii; and carcinoid syndrome; derived from embryonic tissue	Mature teratoma
Calcifications (like benign teratoma); cells from all three germ layers; excellent prognosis in early stages	Immature teratoma
Rare; usually diagnosed at <20 years; ↑ β-hCG	Choriocarcinoma

Name the type of sex cord-stromal tumor characterized below:

Estrogen secretion → precocious puberty; endometrial hyperplasia; Call-Exner bodies; inhibin tumor marker	Granulosa-theca cell tumor
Testosterone secretion → virilization; hirsutism; testosterone tumor marker	Sertoli-Leydig cell tumor

What syndrome is characterized by the triad of ovarian tumor, ascites, and right hydrothorax?	Meig syndrome

Gestational Trophoblastic Neoplasm

What is gestational trophoblastic neoplasm (GTN)?	Rare neoplasms derived from abnormal proliferation of placental tissue

Identify the following three types of hydatidiform moles (molar pregnancies):

Sperm fertilizes an ovum that lacks DNA; karyotype of product is 46XX (paternal DNA duplicates), no fetal parts, often signs of hyperemesis gravidarum, hyperthyroidism (rare)	Complete mole
Two sperms fertilize normal ovum, karyotype of product is 69XXY, fetal parts present	Incomplete mole
Benign GTN that has become malignant, penetrates myometrium, rarely metastasizes	Invasive mole

What are the signs and symptoms consistent with molar pregnancy?	Passage of grape-like vesicles, new-onset HTN <20 weeks GA
What diagnostic abnormalities are typical of molar pregnancy?	hCG >100,000; absence of fetal heart sounds; "snowstorm" on US
What are the four major components of the management of a molar pregnancy?	D&C to evacuate and terminate pregnancy, follow-up with weekly hCG, CXR and LFTs to check for metastasis
What malignant gestational trophoblastic tumor may occur with or after pregnancy (including ectopic, molar, or abortion)?	Choriocarcinoma
What is the characteristic histopathology of choriocarcinoma and how does it spread?	Invasive sheets of trophoblasts associated with hemorrhage and necrosis; metastasizes hematogenously
What is the treatment for choriocarcinoma?	Chemotherapy (almost 100% remission if nonmetastatic)

REPRODUCTIVE ENDOCRINOLOGY

Infertility

What is the definition of infertility?	Inability to conceive after 12 months of unprotected sexual intercourse
What is the incidence of infertility among couples?	15%
What are four major categories of infertility?	1. Male factor (30%) 2. Ovulatory defect (30%) 3. Tubal factor (30%) 4. Unknown/other factors (10%)
What laboratory studies are useful in the evaluation of an infertile couple?	TSH, FSH, and prolactin and semen analysis
What is a normal sperm count in semen analysis?	≥20 million/mL
What are three methods used to establish ovulation?	1. Basal body temperature: should ↑ by 0.5°C (32.9°F) after ovulation occurs 2. Progesterone: 4 ng/mL in luteal phase confirm ovulation 3. Endometrial biopsy: should see secretory phase

How are the uterus and fallopian tubes evaluated in the workup of female factor infertility?	Hysterosalpingography: look for obstruction → if negative → exploratory laparoscopy: look for adhesions, endometriosis
What is the treatment of infertility caused by anovulation?	Clomiphene or FSH

Dysfunctional Uterine Bleeding

Define dysfunctional uterine bleeding:	Anovulatory, abnormal uterine bleeding due to hormonal disruption and not due to organic cause (eg, polyps/cervicitis)
How is dysfunctional uterine bleeding diagnosed?	Diagnosis of exclusion; must rule out organic lesions of reproductive tract, iatrogenic causes, gestational disorders, and coagulopathies
Name two common situations in which dysfunctional uterine bleeding may occur:	1. Extremes of reproductive life: adolescents who have not yet established regular cycles and perimenopausal women 2. After changes in lifestyle: factors such as diet and stress can cause regular cycles to become irregular

Amenorrhea

What is the definition of primary (1°) amenorrhea?	Absence of menses by age 16 despite secondary sexual characteristics
What are the Müllerian structures?	Fallopian tubes, uterus, and upper one-third of vagina (not ovaries)
What are three general causes of 1° amenorrhea?	1. Outflow tract obstruction 2. Ovarian failure 3. Hypothalamic disorder
If the uterus is absent, what test should be ordered in the workup of 1° amenorrhea?	Karyotype
What is the definition of 2° amenorrhea?	Absence of menses ≥6 months in a woman with h/o normal menses

What is the most common cause of 2° amenorrhea?

Pregnancy

Name the cause of 2° amenorrhea described below:

Uterine scarring, adhesions from D&C, CS, or myomectomy

Asherman syndrome

Surgical or obstetrical trauma

Cervical stenosis

Pan-hypopituitarism resulting from pituitary infarction caused by PP shock or hemorrhage

Sheehan syndrome

↑ prolactin production

Prolactinoma

Idiopathic or due to wedge resection of ovary

Premature ovarian failure

Excessive exercising

Hypothalamic etiology

↓ T3/T4 →↑ thyrotropin-releasing hormone (TRH) and prolactin

Hypothyroidism

Chronic anovulation, ↑ LH/FSH ratio; triad of amenorrhea, hirsutism, and obesity

Polycystic ovarian syndrome (PCOS)

Side effect of antipsychotic medications

Drug-induced hyperprolactinemia

Patients with PCOS are at risk for what three conditions?

1. Infertility
2. DM
3. Endometrial hyperplasia/CA

Provide the treatment for the following causes of amenorrhea:

Hypothalamic

Tumor removal, weight gain, stress relief, and exogenous GnRH

Pituitary

Tumor removal, bromocriptine (prolactin inhibitor), and exogenous FSH/LH

Ovarian

PCOS: Clomiphene for fertility, progestin-containing contraception to prevent endometrial hyperplasia, and weight loss to prevent DM

Ovarian failure: OCPs, donor egg

Uterine

Surgery for lysis of adhesions

UROGYNECOLOGY

Pelvic Prolapse

Name four types of pelvic prolapses:	1. Cystocele 2. Rectocele 3. Enterocele 4. Uterine prolapse
What are the risk factors for pelvic organ prolapse?	Childbirth injury, aging, estrogen deficiency, connective tissue weakness, constipation, obesity, and coughing
What are the signs and symptoms of pelvic organ prolapse?	Pressure, organ protrusion, incontinence, dyspareunia, groin pain
How is pelvic organ prolapse diagnosed?	Manual inspection of urethra, vagina, perineum, and anal sphincter
What are nonsurgical management options for pelvic organ prolapse?	Lifestyle changes: stop smoking, lose weight, Kegel exercises, prevent constipation; pessary: intravaginal device to support prolapse
When is surgical treatment a good option for pelvic organ prolapse?	Symptomatic prolapse refractory to pessary

Urinary Incontinence

Provide the name and treatment for each type of incontinence described below:	
Bladder pressure → urethral pressure due to increased abdominal pressure from coughing, sneezing, running	Stress incontinence (usually due to urethral hypermobility ± sphincter dysfunction) **Tx:** Kegel exercises, estrogen therapy, alpha-adrenergic drugs, surgery (Burch, transvaginal tape [TVT])
Overactivity of bladder smooth muscle	Detrusor instability *or* urge incontinence (may be due to neurologic disease or irritation) **Tx:** anticholinergics and timed voiding
Overdistension of bladder	Overflow incontinence **Tx:** alpha-adrenergics, striated muscle relaxants, and self-catheterization

MAKE THE DIAGNOSIS

40-y/o G4P5 female who just delivered twins followed by two whole placentas now has copious vaginal bleeding; PE: ~800 cc blood in 5 min, boggy uterus

Uterine atony

60-y/o postmenopausal, nulliparous, obese female with 5-year h/o HRT presents with vaginal spotting; PE: normal pelvic examination; workup (w/u): abnormal endometrial biopsy

Endometrial cancer

39-y/o G2P1 black female at 28 weeks gestation presents with increasing left lower quadrant (LLQ) tenderness; PE: abdominal tenderness, asymmetric uterine shape; US: 5 cm × 7 cm uterine mass

Submucosal leiomyoma (with red degeneration)

45-y/o female with recent h/o hysterectomy now presents with constant urinary leakage; PE: clear fluid in vaginal vault; w/u: clear fluid, Cr = 15, ⊕ methylene blue test

Vesicovaginal fistula

30-y/o G1P0 obese female at 32 weeks gestation (verified by LMP) presents for her first prenatal visit; PE: fundal height = 37 cm, FHT are within normal limits (WNL); US: AFI = 27 with single intrauterine pregnancy; glucola = 210 mg/dL

Gestational diabetes mellitus (GDM)

23-y/o G1P0 female at 12 weeks gestation presents with vaginal spotting and N/V; PE: 3-cm cervical dilation; US: intrauterine pregnancy with cardiac activity

Inevitable abortion

25-y/o G1P1 female who just delivered a 3500-g baby continues to have vaginal bleeding after delivery of placenta; PE: vaginal laceration dissecting the perineum with an intact anal sphincter

Second-degree laceration

23-y/o nulligravid female with multiple partners presents with abdominal tenderness and fever; PE: cervical motion tenderness, uterine tenderness, no adnexal tenderness, no genital lesions; US: uterus and adnexae are WNL.

Pelvic inflammatory disease (PID)

32-y/o G2P1 female at 37 weeks gestation presents in labor; PE: active phase of first stage of labor; w/u: FHR = 130 bpm, tracing shows shallow symmetrical decelerations in the "mirror image" of each contraction.

Fetal head compression

42-y/o G2P1 Asian female at 10 weeks gestation presents with N/V; PE: ↑ HR, ↑ BP, closed cervical os; w/u: β-hCG = 10,000; US shows "snowstorm" pattern and no IUP; karyotype: 46XX

Complete molar pregnancy

18-y/o sexually active female presents for annual gynecologic examination; PE: red and tender cervix, no uterine or adnexal tenderness; w/u: no growth on culture

Cervicitis from *Chlamydia* infection

68-y/o Caucasian female with h/o ovarian cancer, surgical staging, and taxol/carboplatin therapy 2 years ago now presents with bloating; PE: ascites and weight loss; w/u: CA-125 = 1200

Recurrent ovarian cancer

19-y/o G1P0 black female with twin gestation at 35 weeks gestation presents with headaches and blurred vision; PE: BP = 148/102, facial edema, no abdominal tenderness or hyperreflexia; w/u: 2 protein on urine dipstick

Mild preeclampsia

28-y/o G3P2 female presents at term in labor; PE: fetal head at top of fundus by Leopold maneuvers; US: breech presentation with both feet near fetal head

Frank breech

30-y/o G2P1 female at 34 weeks gestation presented with PTL and has been on $MgSO_4$ for 24 h; PE: lethargy, ↓↓ DTRs; w/u: ECG shows ↑ PR and QT intervals.

Magnesium toxicity (>10 meq/L)

17-y/o G1P1 single female who is 7 months PP now presents with 6-month h/o weight loss, insomnia, and dysphoria; PE: poor attention to personal appearance; w/u: TFTs are WNL.

Postpartum depression

31-y/o nulligravid female with h/o infrequent menses and Type 2 DM presents with infertility; PE: obese, facial hair, female phenotype; w/u: LH/ FSH >3; progesterone challenge test induces menses.

Polycystic ovarian syndrome (PCOS)

18-y/o G1P0 female at 22 weeks gestation presents with persistent N/V; PE: poor skin turgor, dry mucous membranes; w/u: hypochloremic alkalosis; TFT, LFTs, amylase, and lipase are all WNL.

Hyperemesis gravidarum

37-y/o G2P1 black female at 34 weeks gestation who smokes 1/2 ppd presents with painful vaginal bleeding and contractions; PE: ↑ HR, uterine tenderness, blood in vaginal vault

Placental abruption

65-y/o G4P4 female with h/o chronic bronchitis presents with urinary incontinence when coughing or laughing, but denies nocturia; PE: incontinence when asked to cough, cotton swab test = 45°; UA and culture are WNL.

Stress incontinence

24-y/o G1P0 female at 28 weeks gestation presents for a routine US; PE: consistent with 28-week twin gestation; US: same-sex twins sharing one placenta, with polyhydramnios of one amniotic sac and oligohydramnios of the other; fetal weight difference >20%

Twin-to-twin transfusion syndrome

21-y/o female with h/o PID presents with cramping and vaginal spotting; PE: abdominal tenderness; w/u: ⊕ β-hCG; US: empty uterus

Ectopic pregnancy

23-y/o G2P2 female with h/o uncontrolled Type 1 DM presents 1 day after CS with fever; PE: fever = 38.8°C (102°F), uterine tenderness, and malodorous lochi; w/u: WBC = 16,000; UA and urine culture are negative.

Endometritis

39-y/o G2P1 female at 18 weeks gestation presents for routine prenatal care visit; PE: consistent with 18-week pregnancy; w/u: triple screen shows ↓ AFP and estriol, and ↑ β-hCG; US: thickened nuchal skin and short femurs

Down syndrome fetus (increased likelihood)

30-y/o G1P0 Caucasian female at 32 weeks gestation presents with malaise, N/V, and abdominal tenderness; PE: BP = 150/98, RUQ tenderness; w/u: platelets = 70,000, ↑ LFTs; peripheral blood smear shows hemolysis.

HELLP syndrome

36-y/o HIV-positive female with h/o tobacco and heroin use presents with vaginal spotting; PE: cachexia, friable cervix with a mass

Cervical cancer

27-y/o nulligravid female presents with 6-month h/o pelvic pain that increases when she is menstruating; PE: tender left ovary; US: 3-cm left adnexal mass; UA, cultures, and pregnancy test are all negative.

Endometrioma

29-y/o G1P0 female at 31 weeks gestation presents with complaint of leaking clear fluid; she denies contractions, vaginal bleeding, or fevers; PE: sterile speculum examination shows pool of clear fluid in vaginal vault; w/u: nitrazine test is blue.

Preterm premature rupture of membranes (PPROM)

61-y/o G5P5 female with h/o traumatic labor 20 years prior presents with pelvic pressure and urinary frequency; PE: cervix visualized and palpated just behind the introitus

Prolapsed uterus

36-y/o G2P2 female with h/o abdominal hysterectomy for unrelenting postpartum hemorrhage and hypotension (8 months ago) presents with 2° amenorrhea since then; w/u: negative β-hCG, ↓ serum prolactin

Sheehan syndrome

24-y/o G1P0 female at 33 weeks gestation is hospitalized for polyhydramnios of unknown etiology; PE: fundal height greater than dates; w/u: fetal heart tracing shows sinusoidal wave pattern.

Cord prolapsed

32-y/o G3P3 with h/o retained placenta requiring D&C, now at 12 months postpartum with lack of menses since delivery

Asherman syndrome

27-y/o G2P1 with h/o prior cesarean section attempting trial of labor after c-section with change in station from +1 to 2 and loss of uterine tone seen on tocometry and recurrent late decelerations

Uterine rupture

22-y/o G0 attempting pregnancy for 12 months without success. She reports symptoms of headache, vision changes, and galactorrhea. PE: WNL

Pituitary adenoma (prolactin secreting)

17-y/o female presents with vulvar pain and extreme difficulty with placement of a tampon. PE: positive Q-tip test

Vulvar vestibulitis

26-y/o G2P1 female who presents with 1-week history of thin, malodorous discharge, worse after intercourse. Wet mount reveals >20% clue cells.

Bacterial vaginosis

CHAPTER 6

Pediatrics

GENETIC DEFECTS

Name the trisomy in the following
descriptions:

Endocardial cushion defects,
duodenal atresia, Hirschsprung
disease, hypothyroidism, mental
retardation (MR), leukemia,
Alzheimer-like dementia

Trisomy 21(Down syndrome)

Trisomy associated with rocker-
bottom feet and micrognathia

Trisomy 18 (Edward syndrome)

Trisomy associated with
micophthalmia, holoprosencephaly,
polydactyly, microcephaly, and cleft
lip/palate

Trisomy 13 (Patau sydrome)

Most common chromosomal
abnormality

Trisomy 21 (Down syndrome)

What syndrome is characterized by
the karyotype 45, XO?

Turner syndrome

Name five dysmorphic features
associated with Turner syndrome:

1. Lymphedema of the hands and feet
2. Shield-shaped chest
3. Widely spaced nipples
4. Webbed neck
5. Low hair line

Name the common cardiac defects
associated with Turner syndrome:

Coarctation of the aorta, bicuspid aortic
valve, and aortic stenosis

What gonadal abnormality occurs in
100% of Turner patients?

Gonadal dysgenesis

What is the treatment regimen for
Turner patients?

Growth hormone for short stature and
estrogen/progesterone for secondary
sexual development

What is the most common cause of hypogonadism in males?	Klinefelter syndrome (47, XXY)
What are five clinical manifestations of Klinefelter syndrome?	1. Small phallus 2. Small testes (hypospermia) 3. Gynecomastia 4. Increased height 5. Learning disability with normal IQ
What is a Barr body?	An inactivated X chromosome associated with Klinefelter syndrome
What hormone is used to treat Klinefelter syndrome?	Testosterone (improves secondary sexual characteristics and prevents gynecomastia)
What syndrome is associated with uncontrollable appetite and Pickwickian syndrome?	Prader-Willi syndrome
What is the mode of inheritance in Prader-Willi syndrome?	Paternal imprinting
What disease is known as the "happy puppet" syndrome?	Angelman syndrome, due to ataxic gait and tip-toe walk (patients also have severe MR and episodes of uncontrollable laughter)
What is the mode of inheritance in Angelman syndrome?	Maternal imprinting
What inherited syndrome, characterized by severe mental retardation, is caused by trinucleotide repeats?	Fragile X syndrome

CONGENITAL HEART DISEASE

Name the five congenitally acquired cyanotic heart lesions:	"12345" 1. Truncus arteriosus (**one** arterial vessel overrides ventricles) 2. Transposition of the great vessels (**two** arteries are switched) 3. **Tri**cuspid atresia 4. **Tetra**logy of Fallot 5. Total anomolous pulmonary venous return (**five** words)

Name the cyanotic heart lesion
described in the following situations:

Most common cyanotic lesion
presenting in the first 2 weeks of life

Transposition of the great vessels

"Boot-shaped heart" and decreased
pulmonary vascular markings on
chest x-ray CXR

Tetralogy of Fallot

Cardiomegaly and an "egg-shaped
silhouette" on CXR

Transposition of the great vessels

Treatment consists of arterial switch
performed in the first 2 weeks of life.

Transposition of the great vessels (left
ventricle will decompensate if procedure
is delayed >2 weeks)

Cardiac defect wherein pulmonary
venous blood is directed to the
right atrium

Total/parital anomalous pulmonary
venous return

Characterized by periods of
increased right outflow obstruction
that cause cyanosis by increasing
right-to-left shunting

Tetralogy of Fallot ("tet spells")

Name the four defects in tetralogy
of Fallot:

"PROVe"
1. **P**ulmonic stenosis
2. **R**ight ventricular hypertrophy
3. "**O**verriding aorta"
4. **V**entricular septal defect (VSD)

What congenital heart lesion is defined
as tricuspid valve displacement into
the right ventricle?

Ebstein anomaly

Which maternally ingested drug is
associated with Ebstein anomaly
in the child?

Lithium

Name three acyanotic heart lesions:

1. VS**D**
2. Atrial septal defect (AS**D**)
3. Patent ductus arteriosus (PD**A**)—all
   contain the letter "**D**".

What is the most common congenital
heart defect?

VSD

What is the feared complication of a
large, untreated VSD?

Eisenmenger syndrome

What results from a deficiency of the
endocardial cushion?

Atrioventricular (AV) canal defect—
ostium primum ASD and inlet VSD

What congenital infection is associated
with a PDA?

Rubell-**A**→PD**A**

What is the mode of inheritance in hypertrophic cardiomyopathy?	Autosomal dominant
What are the prominent symptoms in hypertrophic cardiomyopathy?	Chest pain, dyspnea on exertion, and syncope (common cause of sudden cardiac death in athletes)

Name the bradyarrhythmia in the following ECG descriptions:

Prolonged PR interval with a regular rhythm	First-degree heart block
Progressive prolongation of the PR interval until a QRS complex is missed	Mobitz type I (Wenckebach)
Sudden disruption in AV conduction with no progressive prolongation of the PR interval	Mobitz type II
"Complete AV dissociation"	Third-degree heart block
What are the most common causes of sinus tachycardia?	Fever, dehydration, exercise, and anemia
Name the key ECG manifestation of Wolff-Parkinson-White syndrome:	Delta wave (caused by preexcitation of the ventricle via an accessory pathway)
Which antiarrhythmic drug is contraindicated in Wolff-Parkinson-White syndrome?	Digoxin (by slowing the AV node, an accessory pathway can repolarize and potentially create a reentrant circuit)

DEVELOPMENT

Milestones

At what age is an average child expected to:

Walk	12 months
Run	18 months
Display stranger anxiety	7 months
Use a pincer grasp	9 months (the number "9" is made when the pincer grasp is held upside down)
Hold their head up	3 months
Sit up without support	6 months
Say their first word	12 months (1 word at 1 year)
Use two-word combinations	24 months (2 words at 2 years)
Use three-word sentences	36 months (3 words at 3 years)
Crawl	9 months

| Walk up and down stairs | 24 months |
| Feed himself/herself with utensils | 18 months |

List the sequence of events that occur in female puberty:	Thelarche (breast development)
	Pubarche (development of pubic hair)
	Growth spurt
	Menarche (first menstrual period)

List the sequence of events that occur in male puberty:	Testicular enlargement
	Pubarche
	Penile enlargement
	Growth spurt

Name the Tanner stage:

| Breast bud development and enlargement of areolar diameter | Tanner stage II |
| Increased darkening of scrotal skin | Tanner stage IV |

Vaccinations

| Name the current recommended childhood vaccinations: | Hepatitis B vaccine, diphtheria toxoid, tetanus toxoid, pertussis vaccine, Haemophilus influenzae type b (Hib) vaccine, pneumococcal vaccine, poliomyelitis vaccine, rotavirus vaccine, influenza vaccine, measles vaccine, mumps vaccine, rubella vaccine, varicella vaccine, Hepatitis A vaccine, meningococcal vaccine, HPV vaccine (girls only) |

| What vaccine is administered shortly after birth? | Hepatitis B virus vaccine (hepatitis **B** at **B**irth) |

List the vaccination regimen for the following organisms:

Hepatitis B	Birth/1-2 months, 6-18 months
Polio	2 months, 4 months, 6-18 months/ 4-6 years
Measles, mumps, and rubella (MMR)	12-15 months, 4-6 years
Diphtheria-tetanus-pertussis (DTaP)	2 months, 4 months, 6 months, 15-18 months/4-6 years; tetanus booster required every 5-10 years
Haemophilus influenzae type b (Hib)	2 months, 4 months, 6 months, 12-15 months
Pneumococcus (PCV)	2 months, 4 months, 6 months, 12-15 months

What type of polio vaccine is recommended in the United States?	Inactivated polio vaccine (IPV) (the oral vaccine [OPV] is the number one cause of polio in the US)
What age must a child be in order to receive a varicella vaccination?	>12 months

Name the vaccination(s):

Contraindicated in immunocompromised patients	MMR, varicella, and oral polio vaccine (OPV)
Containing egg protein	MMR and influenza
Required in asplenic patients	Pneumococcal, meningococcal, and Hib vaccines (these are the encapsulated organism vaccines)
Contraindicated in patients with progressive neurologic disorders or encephalopathy within 7 days of administration	DTaP (the pertussis component is associated with seizures)
Conjugated vaccinations	Hib, meningococcal, and pneumococcal vaccines

Failure to Thrive

Define failure to thrive (FTT):	FTT is a condition in which a child's weight or height is less than the third to fifth percentile for age or has fallen across two major percentiles.
List the major risk factors of FTT:	1. Low socioeconomic status 2. Low maternal age 3. Low birth weight 4. Caregiver neglect 5. Pathologic disease
What are common organic causes of FTT?	1. Congenital heart disease 2. Cystic fibrosis 3. Celiac disease 4. Pyloric stenosis 5. Infection 6. Gastroesophageal reflux

IMMUNODEFIENCY SYNDROMES

At what age do T-cell immunodeficiencies present and what type of infections occur?	1-3 months; broad range infections (fungal, bacterial, viral)

List two of the most common T-cell deficiency syndromes:	1. DiGeorge syndrome 2. Ataxia-telangiectasia
What is the embryonal deformity in DiGeorge syndrome?	Agenesis of the third and fourth pharyngeal pouch (responsible for the development of the thymus and parathyroid gland)
List the clinical manifestations of DiGeorge syndrome:	**CATCH-22** **C**ardiac anomalies (tetralogy of Fallot, interrupted aortic arch, and vascular rings) **A**bnormal facies **T**hymic hypoplasia **C**left palate **H**ypocalcemia **22** (chromosome 22q11 microdeletion)
List the characteristics of ataxia-telangiectasia:	Cerebellar ataxia, oculocutaneous telangiectasia, decreased T-cell function, and low antibody levels (considered to be combined immunodeficiency in some texts)
At what age do B-cell deficiency syndromes typically present?	6 months (maternal antibodies protect infant up to this age)
What type of infections occur in B-cell deficiency syndromes?	Recurrent upper respiratory infections and bacteremia caused by encapsulated organisms
Name the three most common B-cell deficiency syndromes:	1. X-linked agammaglobulinema 2. Common variable immunodefiency 3. Selective IgA deficiency
Name the disease characterized by a total lack of antibody production:	X-linked (Bruton) agammaglobulinemia
Name the disease characterized by recurrent respiratory, GI, and urinary tract infections:	Selective IgA deficiency
List the two most common combined B- and T-cell immunodeficiency syndromes:	1. Severe combined immunodeficiency disease (SCID) 2. Wiskott-Aldrich syndrome
What is the treatment of SCID?	Bone marrow transplantation is curative.

List the clinical manifestations of Wiskott-Aldrich syndrome:	**WATER** **W**—↓ IgM (W upside down) ↑ IgA **T**hrombocytopenia **E**czema **R**ecurrent infections
What are the clinical manifestations of phagocytic immunodeficiency syndromes?	Poor wound healing, abscess formation, and granulomas
Name the two most common phagocytic syndromes:	1. Chronic granulomatous disease 2. Chediak-Higashi syndrome
What is the mode of inheritance in chronic granulomatous disease?	X-linked recessive
What chemical process are patients afflicted with chronic granulomatous disease unable to perform?	Oxidative burst that produces hydrogen peroxide
What is the mode of inheritance in Chediak-Higashi syndrome and what is the defective immunological process?	Autosomal recessive and neutrophil chemotaxis
What is the oculocutaneous manifestation of Chediak-Higashi syndrome?	Albinism

CHILD ABUSE

Name the finding(s) suggestive of abuse in the following scenarios:	
Cutaneous visual examination	Ecchymoses of varying age and pattern injuries (iron or cigarette burns, immersion burns, belt markings)
Ocular examination	Retinal hemorrhages (shaken baby syndrome)
Radiologic film	Spiral fractures
Genitourinary examination	Sexually transmitted diseases, genital trauma
Head CT scan	Subdural hemorrhage (shaken baby syndrome)

Cerebral Palsy

What defines a nonprogressive, nonhereditary disorder of movement and posture?	Cerebral palsy (CP)
List the risk factors of CP:	1. Prematurity 2. MR 3. Low birth weight 4. Fetal malformation 5. Neonatal seizures 6. Neonatal cerebral hemorrhage 7. Perinatal asphyxia
What is the most frequent presenting sign of CP?	Delayed motor development (often missed until child fails to meet developmental milestones)
What percentage of CP patients display MR?	About 50% (not all have MR)
What is the most common form of CP?	Pyramidal (characterized by spasticity in all affected limbs)
What is the treatment of CP?	Benzodiazepines, dantrolene, and baclofen (goal is to reduce spasticity)

Febrile Seizures

What defines a non-epileptic seizure in children 6 months-5 years of age associated with fevers?	Febrile seizures
What is the cause of febrile seizures?	The rapidity of fever onset, not the absolute temperature, is the determining factor.
Simple or Complex Febrile Seizure?	
Duration <15 min	Simple
More than one seizure in a 24-h period	Complex
Necessitates a lumbar puncture, laboratory studies, EEG and CT/MRI	Complex
Characterized by a generalized seizure	Simple (complex seizures tend to be focal)
Associated with a 2% risk of epilepsy	Simple (risk in general population without febrile seizures is 1%)

NEONATOLOGY

What determines the Apgar score?

APGAR

Appearance (blue/pale, pink trunk, all pink)

Pulse (0, <100, >100)

Grimace with stimulation (0, grimace, grimace and cough)

Activity (limp, some, active)

Respiratory effort (0, irregular, regular)

Determine the Apgar score:

Newborn with a pink trunk, heart rate of 50, a grimace and cough when stimulated, strong muscle tone, and an irregular respiratory effort

7

A blue newborn with a heart rate of 30, a grimace when stimulated, appears limp, and has no respiratory effort

2

Name the organism responsible for the congenital infection in the following clinical scenarios:

A 3-wk/o female infant found to have leukocoria (absent red reflex), a continuous machine-like murmur, "blueberry muffin" skin and "salt and pepper" retinitis

RubellA—PDA

A 1-mo/o male found to have periventricular calcifications on head MRI, hepatosplenomegaly, chorioretinitis, and a left inguinal hernia

Cytomegalovirus

A 3-d/o male found to have skin vesicles and keratoconjunctivitis

Herpes simplex virus

A 2-wk/o female found to have osteochondritis, periostitis, a maculopapular rash, and the "snuffles"

Treponema pallidum

A 1-wk/o male found to have generalized calcifications on head MRI and chorioretinitis

Toxoplasma gondii

A 16-mo/o infant found to have sensorineural hearing loss

RuBELLa—children with congenital rubella cannot hear the BELL.

What HIV serological marker is used to detect the HIV status in an infant of a HIV-positive mother?	HIV DNA PCR
What three organisms are the most likely causes of neonatal sepsis?	**GEL** 1. Group B streptococci 2. *E. coli* 3. *Listeria monocytogenes*
What is the treatment regimen for a neonate with suspected sepsis?	Ampicillin and gentamicin for 7 days
What is the most common cause of respiratory failure in a premature newborn?	Respiratory distress syndrome (RDS)
What is the pathogenesis of RDS?	Lack of adequate surfactant production causing alveolar collapse
What is the typical presentation of RDS?	Tachypnea, grunting, retractions, and nasal flaring in the first few hours of life
What is the typical course of RDS?	Progressive worsening and pending respiratory failure in the first 48-72 hours of life
What are the characteristic findings on CXR of RDS?	Diffuse atelectasis and a ground-glass appearance
What is the treatment of RDS?	Usually requires intubation and surfactant administration
What are the complications of treatment of RDS?	Bronchopulmonary dysplasia, retinopathy of prematurity, and barotrauma from mechanical ventilation
What is physiologic jaundice?	Transient, unconjugated hyperbilirubinemia caused by large bilirubin load that overwhelms a maturing liver system
What three features differentiate physiologic jaundice from pathologic jaundice?	The following three are all features of pathologic jaundice: 1. Hyperbilirubinemia in the first 24 h 2. Prolonged jaundice 3. Conjugated hyperbilirubinemia
Name the fatal complication of neonatal hyperbilirubinemia:	Kernicterus (bilirubin staining of the basal ganglia, pons, and cerebellum)

Name the two therapies available for severe jaundice:	1. Phototherapy 2. Exchange transfusion
What is the pathognomonic radiographic finding in patients with necrotizing enterocolitis?	Pneumatosis intestinalis

Name the likely congenital anomaly in the following clinical scenarios:

Neonate with inability to feed, excessive salivation, and recurrent aspiration pneumonia with a polyhydramniotic mother	Tracheoesophageal fistula
Neonate with bilious emesis and a "double-bubble" sign on abdominal radiograph	Duodenal atresia
Neonate born with abdominal viscera herniating through the umbilicus, contained in a sac	Omphalocele (gastroschisis contains no sac), omphalocele associated with other congenital anomalies

INFECTIOUS DISEASE

Name the complications of Group A streptococcal infections:	Peritonsillar abscess, retropharyngeal abscess, rheumatic fever, poststreptococcal glomerulonephritis
Which complication is not avoided with antibiotic treatment?	Poststreptococcal glomerulonephritis (PSGN)
Name the four clinical manifestations of PSGN:	Hematuria, oliguria, hypertension, and edema
What are the major manifestations of acute rheumatic fever?	**JONES** Joints (migratory polyarthritis) O—pancarditis ("♥" is in the shape of a heart) Subcutaneous Nodules Erythema marginatum Sydenham chorea
What is the critical determinant of morbidity in acute rheumatic fever?	Mitral and aortic valve stenosis/ regurgitation

Name the viral exanthem associated with
the following clinical manifestations:

Cough, coryza, conjunctivitis	Measles
Fever with a vesicular rash at different stages	Varicella (chickenpox)
Maculopapular rash, febrile seizures, and HHV-6 infection	Roseola infantum

"Slapped-cheek" appearance with
parvovirus B19 infection — Erythema infectiosum (fifth disease)

Painful ulcers on the tongue and oral
mucosa and a maculopapular rash
on the distal limbs and buttocks — Hand, foot, and mouth (and butt)
disease

What is included in the differential
diagnosis for upper airway obstruction? — Foreign body aspiration, croup,
epiglottitis, retropharyngeal abscess,
bacterial tracheitis, angioedema

Croup or epiglottitis?

Most commonly caused by parainfluenza virus infection	Croup
Presents with high fever, "sniffing-dog" position, toxic appearance, and drooling	Epiglottitis
Very rare due to the Hib vaccination	Epiglottitis
Responds to racemic epinephrine	Croup
Requires emergent endotracheal intubation	Epiglottitis
"Steeple sign" on anteroposterior (AP) neck films	Croup (think of a Group of people going to the steeple)
Presents with inspiratory stridor and a "barky" cough	Croup

What three bacteria most frequently
cause otitis media (OM)? — *S. pneumonia*
Non-typeable *H. influenza*
Moraxella catarrhalis

What are the findings of OM on
otologic examination? — Bulging tympanic membrane (TM),
loss of TM light reflex, decreased
mobility of the TM on pneumatic
otoscopy

What is the typical treatment for OM? — High-dose amoxicillin (80-90 mg/kg/d)
for 10 days, resistant organisms require
amoxicillin-clavulanic acid (Augmentin)

What pathogen causes most cases of bronchiolitis?	Respiratory syncytial virus
What is the recommended treatment for a neonate with bacterial meningitis?	Ampicillin and cefotaxime (older children—vancomycin and ceftriaxone)

Specify the organism associated with gastroenteritis in the following cases:

Neurologic symptoms of seizures, mental status changes, and lethargy	*Shigella*
Capable of causing sepsis and meningitis	*Salmonella*
Most common nonbacterial agent	Rotavirus (incidence now decreasing with vaccination)
"Pseudoappendicitis" picture	*Yersinia*
Hemolytic uremic syndrome	*E. coli* O157:H7 (90% of cases)

NEPHROLOGY

What is the most frequent clinical sign of vesicoureteral reflux?	Recurrent UTIs
What is the diagnostic test of choice in vesicoureteral reflux?	Voiding cystourethrogram (VCUG)
Name the most common penile congenital anomaly:	Hypospadias
What are the two major complications of cryptorchidism?	1. Impaired sperm production 2. Increased risk of malignancy
Name the four characteristics of nephrotic syndrome:	1. Proteinuria 2. Hypoalbuminemia 3. Hyperlipidemia 4. Edema
What is the most common cause of nephrotic syndrome and what is the treatment?	Minimal change disease; steroids (best prognosis)
What is the hallmark of glomerulonephritis?	Hematuria

Name the glomerulonephritis in the
following situations:

Hematuria preceded by pharyngitis 2 weeks prior	Acute poststreptococcal glomerulonephritis (most common)
Hematuria with an insidious regression to renal failure and encephalopathy	Rapidly progressive glomerulonephritis
Palpable purpura on the lower limbs and buttocks followed by abdominal pain and hematuria	Henoch-Schonlein purpura
Nephritic clinical picture accompanied by sensorineural hearing loss	Alport syndrome
Elevated ASO titer and low complement C3 levels	Acute poststreptococcal glomerulonephritis

GASTROENTEROLOGY

Name the gastrointestinal disease
characterized by the following
descriptions:

Most common indication for surgical intervention	Appendicitis
Most common cause of bowel obstruction in children <2 years	Intussusception
Characterized by projectile, non-bilious vomiting in firstborn males 2-5 weeks of age	Pyloric stenosis
Air contrast enema is diagnostic and therapeutic.	Intussusception
Physical examination reveals an olive-shaped, mobile, non-tender mass.	Pyloric stenosis
Manifests as crampy, abdominal pain with emesis and bloody, mucousy stool ("currant jelly" stool)	Intussusception
Presents as painless, rectal bleeding	Meckel diverticulum
Failure of ganglionic cell migration	Hirschsprung disease
Arises from "lead points" and is described as a "sausage-like mass" on examination	Intussusception

Diagnosis requires a technetium pertechnetate scan that detects ectopic gastric musoca.	Meckel diverticulum
Diagnosis requires ultrasound and treatment is by surgical pylorotomy.	Pyloric stenosis
Typically presents as bilious emesis in a child <1 month of age and is diagnosed by an upper GI series	Malrotation
Risk factors include Meckel diverticulum, intestinal lymphoma, Henoch-Schonlein purpura, celiac disease, cystic fibrosis, and infection.	Intussusception (all can act as potential "lead points")

Name the major characteristics of Meckel diverticulum:	**Rule of 2s**
	Males are affected **2** times as often as females
	2 feet from the ileocecal valve
	2 types of ectopic mucosa (gastric or pancreatic)
	2% of population
	2 months to **2** years of age

ENDOCRINOLOGY

What disease results from the lack of insulin production by B cells in the pancreas?	Insulin-dependent diabetes mellitus (type 1)
What are the characteristics of diabetic ketoacidosis (DKA)?	Hyperglycemia, ketoacidosis, dehydration, and lethargy
What is the typical presentation of a type 1 diabetic patient?	Polyuria, polydypsia, fatigue, and abdominal pain
What three screening tests should be performed regularly in the pediatric patient with type 1 diabetes?	1. Urine screening for microalbuminemia 2. Ophthalmologic examination for retinopathy 3. Lipid profile for hyperlipidemia
What are the treatment goals for DKA?	Fluid resuscitation, insulin therapy, and electrolyte management
What is the most feared complication in the treatment of a patient in DKA?	Cerebral edema (insulin drives glucose into cells thus altering osmotic pressure)

**Constitutional delay or familial
short stature?**

Normal growth velocity at or below the fifth percentile	Constitutional delay
Growth curves fall below the fifth percentile with abnormal growth velocity	Familial short stature
Delay in bone age	Constitutional delay
Puberty is typically delayed	Constitutional delay
Normal bone age	Familial short stature

List the six most common pathologic causes of short stature:	1. Growth hormone deficiency 2. Primary hypothyroidism 3. Cushing disease 4. Chronic systemic disease 5. Psychosocial deprivation 6. Turner syndrome
What congenital hormonal deficiency can cause severe mental retardation?	Congenital hypothyroidism
What is the most common enzyme deficiency in congenital adrenal hyperplasia?	21-hydroxylase deficiency
What are the clinical manifestations of 21-hydroxylase deficiency?	Ambiguous genitalia, hyponatremia and hyperkalemia (from lack of aldosterone), and hypoglycemia (from insufficient cortisol)
The elevation of what hormone is diagnostic for 21-hydroxylase deficiency?	17-hydroxyprogesterone
What hormonal therapy is used to treat 21-hydroxylase deficiency?	Glucocorticoids (for suppression of androgen production) +/− mineralocorticoids (for electrolyte balance)

HEMATOLOGY

**Name the cause of anemia in the
following descriptions:**

Most common cause of anemia in the pediatric population	Iron deficiency
Patients present with bone/chest pain, dactylitis, priapism or strokes	Sickle cell disease

Has an autosomal dominant mode of inheritance and is diagnosed by a positive osmotic fragility test	Hereditary spherocytosis
Characterized by a depletion of NADPH and an inability to replenish reduced glutathione	Glucose-6-phosphate dehydrogenase deficiency (G6PD)
Inherited hemolytic anemia caused by malformation or malfunction of globin subunits of the hemoglobin molecule	Thalassemia
Treatment of acute symptoms consists of oxygen, analgesia, antibiotics, and exchange transfusion	Sickle cell disease
Complete absence of all 4-alpha-globin genes	Bart's hemoglobin
Absence of 3-alpha-globin genes	Hemoglobin H disease
Characterized by high levels of hemoglobin F	Beta-thalassemia major (F major)
Characterized by high levels of hemoglobin A_2	Beta-thalassemia minor (A minor)
History of drinking >24 ounces of cow's milk per day or transition to cow's milk before 12 months	Iron deficiency anemia
Presents with peripheral neuropathy and paresthesias and causes posterior column spinal degeneration	Vitamin B_{12} deficiency
Typically found on newborn screen, although may present after 4 months of age when hemoglobin F levels begin to decline	Sickle cell disease
X-linked recessive disease that presents during oxidative stress caused by fava beans or drug exposure (dapsone, sulfonamides, and antimalarials)	G6PD
Patients are at greatest risk for infection and sepsis from *H. influenza* and *S. pneumoniae*	Sickle cell disease (spleen may be compromised due to autoinfarction)
Caused by a defective DNA repair mechanism and presents with hyperpigmentation and café-au-lait spots	Fanconi anemia

Name the complication of sickle cell disease described in the following:

Caused by infarction and hemolysis of lung tissue	Acute chest syndrome
Painful swelling of the hands and feet	Dactylitis
Potentially fatal complication typically induced by parvovirus B19 infection	Aplastic crisis (must check reticulocyte count in sickle patients)
Complication that causes pain, priapism, gallbladder disease, chronic renal failure, splenic infarction, and avascular necrosis of the femoral head	Vasoocclusive episode
Sickle cells cause microvascular obstruction and lead to fibrosis of the spleen	Autoinfarction (increased susceptibility of infection with encapsulated organisms)

Name the coagulation disorder(s) in the following description:

X-linked recessive disease caused by a deficiency in factor VIII	Hemophilia A
X-linked recessive disease caused by a deficiency in factor IX	Hemophilia B
Treated with desmopressin acetate (DDAVP)	von Willebrand disease and hemophilia A (DDAVP causes release of factor VIII and vWF from endothelial cells)
Bleeding sites are from mucous membranes, skin, and vagina during menstruation	von Willebrand disease
Bleeding causes hemarthroses and intramuscular bleeds	Hemophilia A and B
Increase in PTT with normal PT and platelet aggregation	Hemophilia A/B and von Willebrand disease

PULMONOLOGY

What common disease is described as a reversible airway obstruction with accompanying bronchial hypersensitivity?	Asthma

Specify the recommended treatment regimen in the following asthma cases:

Patient with symptoms 3 d/wk	Low-dose inhaled corticosteroids (mild persistent)
Patient with symptoms <2 d/wk	Short-acting inhaled beta-2 agonist as needed (mild intermittent)
Patient with symptoms continually during the day and frequently at night	High-dose inhaled corticosteroids and a long-acting beta-2 agonist (severe persistent)
Patient with symptoms daily and several times a week at night	Low-dose inhaled corticosteroids and a long-acting beta-2 agonist or medium-dose inhaled corticosteroids (moderate persistent)
Patient presenting to the ER with an acute exacerbation	ABC's, nebulized beta-2 agonist, nebulized anticholinergic, steroid load +/− supplemental oxygen. If severly ill, consider epinephrine SC, magnesium sulfate or terbutaline.

What disease is caused by a defect in the chloride channel on epithelial cells?	Cystic fibrosis (CF)
Name the mode of inheritance and the chromosome responsible for CF:	Autosomal recessive on chromosome 7 (cystic fibrosis)
What gastrointestinal manifestation in the neonate is pathognomonic for CF?	Meconium ileus (intestinal obstruction following inspissation of meconium)
What is the most common manifestation of CF in infants and children?	Failure to thrive

Name the most common clinical manifestations of CF in the following organ systems:

Respiratory	1. Nasal polyps 2. Sinusitis 3. Bacterial pneumonia 4. Digital clubbing 5. Cough 6. Hemoptysis
Gastrointestinal	Pancreatic insufficieny (causing malabsorption, diarrhea, and failure to thrive), diabetes, rectal prolapse, and meconium ileus

Hepatobiliary	Neonatal jaundice, portal hypertension, and cirrhosis
Reproductive	Impaired fertility in males
Name the diagnostic test of choice in CF:	Sweat chloride test
What is the recommended treatment for CF?	Inhaled respiratory treatments, chest physiotherapy, pancreatic enzymes, vitamins, and antibiotics (as needed)

ONCOLOGY

What is the most common childhood malignancy?	Leukemia (acute lymphocytic leukemia is the most common)
Acute myelogenous leukemia (AML) or acute lymphocytic leukemia (ALL)?	
African American male of any age	AML
White male, 3-5 years of age	ALL
Name the (AML) subtype associated with the following:	
Disseminated intravascular coagulation	M3 (3 words, acute promyelocytic leukemia)
CNS involvement and gingival hyperplasia	M5
What is the typical initial presentation of a patient with leukemia?	Malaise, fever, bruising, and weight loss
What are the typical late presenting signs of leukemia?	Bone pain and arthralgia
The cluster of petechiae, pallor, ecchymoses, and fever in a patient with a history of leukemia is evidence of what pathophysiologic process?	Bone marrow failure
What is the treatment for leukemia?	Steroids, vincristine, intrathecal methotrexate, and asparaginase
What is the most common solid tumor and the second most common malignancy in childhood?	CNS tumors
Where do CNS tumors typically occur?	Infratentorial (cerebellum, midbrain, brainstem) in patients 1-11 years old, supratentorial in patients <1 and >11

Name the clinical manifestations of infratentorial tumors:	Truncal ataxia, coordination/gait disturbances, and head tilt (due to cranial nerve palsies)
What are the symptoms of increased intracranial pressure (ICP)?	Headaches, vomiting, and lethargy
What are the signs of increased ICP?	Hydrocephalus, papilledema, and Cushing triad (hypertension, bradycardia, Cheyne-Stokes respirations—all late findings)

Non-Hodgkin lymphoma or Hodgkin disease?

Represents 60% of pediatric lymphomas	Non-Hodgkin lymphoma
Bimodal distribution of age (14-35 years and 55-74 years)	Hodgkin disease
Diagnosed by the identification of Reed-Sternberg cells in cancerous tissue	Hodgkin disease
Presents with compression symptoms as tumor cells rapidly proliferate	Non-Hodgkin lymphoma
Most commonly presents with painless, firm lymphadenopathy	Hodgkin disease
Peak incidence between the ages of 7 and 11	Non-Hodgkin lymphoma

Name the malignancy of primitive neural crest cells of the adrenal medulla and sympathetic ganglia:	Neuroblastoma
What body region do neuroblastomas most commonly arise from?	Abdomen
What two diagnostic tests provide the definitive diagnosis of neuroblastoma?	Elevated urinary catecholamines and pathological identification of tumor tissue
What clinical manifestations may occur in patients with Wilms tumor associated with other syndromes?	**WAGR** **W**ilms tumor (asymptomatic flank mass) **A**niridia Ambiguous **G**enitalia Mental **R**etardation

Ewing sarcoma or osteosarcoma?

Occurs on the midshaft of bones	Ewing sarcoma (osteosarcoma occurs on the metaphysis)
More likely to have classic "sunburst appearance" on radiograph	Osteosarcoma
Malignant tumor of mesenchymal cells	Osteosarcoma
Undifferentiated small round blue cells	Ewing sarcoma
Surgery and radiation therapy are effective.	Ewing sarcoma (osteosarcoma does not respond to radiation)
20% with metastases at diagnosis	Osteosarcoma and Ewing sarcoma

RHEUMATOLOGY

What pediatric disease is characterized by joint pain, fatigue, rash, lymphadenopathy, and failure to thrive?	Juvenile idiopathic arthritis (JIA)
What laboratory marker indicates an increased risk of uveitis in patients with JIA?	(+) ANA
What is the treatment for JIA?	Anti-inflammatory drugs, immunosuppressive therapy, and physical therapy
What disease is characterized by Gottren papules, violaceous dermatitis, and proximal muscle weakness?	Dermatomyositis
What laboratory value is significantly increased in patients with dermatomyositis?	Serum creatinine kinase

Name the vasculitide associated with the following descriptions:

Positive c-ANCA	Wegener granulomatosis
Palpable purpura, abdominal pain, and hematuria	Henoch-Schonlein purpura

Recurrent upper and lower respiratory tract infections	Wegener granulomatosis
Treated with IVIG and aspirin	Kawasaki disease
Treated with corticosteroids and cyclophosphamide	Wegener granulomatosis
Coronary artery aneurysms are the most concerning complication	Kawasaki disease
What are the clinical manifestations of Kawasaki disease?	**My HEART** **My**—**M**ucous membrane changes (fissured lips and "strawberry tongue") **H**ands and extremity changes (erythema, desquamation, and edema) **E**ye changes (conjunctivitis with limbic sparing) **A**denopathy (cervical, at least 1.5 cm) **R**ash (often in groin area, polymorphous) **T**emperature (>101.4°F for 5 days)

NEUROLOGY

What neurological defect is diagnosed by an increased maternal serum alpha-fetoprotein level?	Neural tube defect
What mineral supplement, when taken by a pregnant mother, can reduce the incidence of neural tube defects?	Folic acid
What type of seizure presents in children <10 years of age?	Absence seizures
Name the EEG pattern that is diagnostic of absence seizures:	Three-per-second spike and wave pattern
What seizure, occuring in children between 2 and 7 months of age, manifests as extensor-flexor spasms occuring up to 100 times in a day?	Infantile spasms
Name the EEG pattern that is diagnostic of infantile spasms:	Hypsarrhythmia (chaotic pattern)

Name the phakomatosis with the
following cutaneous manifestations:

Café-au-lait spots (hyperpigmented   Neurofibromatosis type 1
macules)   (von Recklinghausen disease)

Ash-leaf spots (hypopigmented   Tuberous sclerosis
macules)

Port-wine stains distributed   Sturge-Weber disease
on trigeminal nerve V_1

MISCELLANEOUS

At what age does an average pediatric   1 year
patient triple their birth weight?

What criterion must be met before   Child must be 1 year of age and
a child can ride face forward   20 lb.
in a car seat?

What vitamin supplement must a child   Vitamin D
receive that is strictly breast-fed?

What is the differential diagnosis for   Retinoblastoma, retinopathy of
an infant with leukocoria (lack of a   prematurity, and congenital cataracts
red reflex)?

What is a positive Barlow test?   Posterior-superior dislocation of the hip
with positive pressure (occurs in
developmental hip dysplasia)

What is Ortolani manuever?   Click on hip abduction (occurs in
developmental hip dysplasia)

Name the pathologic cause of
a limp in the following clinical
scenarios:

Obese, adolescent male with referred   Slipped capital femoral epiphysis
pain to the knee   (SCFE)

Painless limp in a 5-year-old child   Legg-Calve-Perthes disease
caused by avascular necrosis of the
femoral head

12-year-old with tibial tuberosity point   Osgood-Schlatter disease
tenderness

What radiographic view is optimal to diagnose SCFE?

Frog-leg lateral view (demonstrates epiphyseal displacement)

Name the organism most likely responsible for osteomyelitis in the following situations:

Most common cause of osteomyelitis

S. aureus

Sickle cell disease

Salmonella

Common in puncture wounds through the sole of a shoe

Pseudomonas aeruginosa

MAKE THE DIAGNOSIS

Newborn infant presents with tachypnea and poor feeding tolerance; continuous machine-like murmur on examination

Patent ductus arteriosus

1-wk/o infant in NICU found to have low set ears, flat occiput, simian crease, small mouth, and protruding tongue; holosystolic murmur on PE

Trisomy 21 (Down syndrome)

1-wk/o infant presents with positive hip click and dislocation of the hip with posterior pressure on routine newborn examination

Developmental hip dysplasia

2-y/o presents with sudden-onset dyspnea and respiratory distress; PE reveals decreased breath sounds on the right side.

Foreign body aspiration

13-y/o presents with fever, emesis, and diffuse periumbilical pain that has localized to the RLQ; PE reveals guarding, tenderness, and positive psoas and obturator signs.

Appendicitis

4-mo/o presents with pallor; PE reveals splenomegaly and a II/VI systolic ejection murmur; Hgb electrophoresis shows high Hgb S concentration.

Sickle cell disease

2-y/o presents with 2-day h/o of non-bloody, watery diarrhea, and vomiting; child attends daycare; PE shows mild dehydration but is otherwise normal.

Viral gastroenteritis

8-y/o presents with painful purpura after jumping on a trampoline; PE reveals palpable purpura on the legs and buttocks with mild abdominal discomfort on examination.

Henoch-Schonlein purpura

5-y/o male with h/o hemarthrosis and subcutaneous bleeding; prolonged PTT and low factor VIII

Hemophilia A

Newborn with h/o trisomy 21 and in utero polyhydramnios presents with bilious emesis; Abdominal x-ray shows "double-bubble" sign.

Duodenal atresia

8-y/o with a h/o IDDM presents with abdominal pain and N/V; PE reveals tachycardia; ABG shows acidosis; urine is positive for ketones.

Diabetic ketoacidosis

13-y/o presents with joint pain and fevers; PE reveals a salmon-colored rash and lymphadenopathy; high WBC and ESR

Juvenile idiopathic arthritis

8-y/o with h/o sickle cell disease presents with severe abdominal pain precipitated by N/V.

Vasoocclusive pain episode

1-y/o presents with irritability and crampy, intermittent abdominal pain with diarrhea; stools are guiac positive; PE reveals tubular, "sausage-like mass."

Intussusception

5-y/o presents with recurrent URI and diarrhea; PE shows nasal polyps, failure to thrive; sweat chloride test is >60 mmol/L.

Cystic fibrosis

14-y/o male presents with gynecomastia; PE reveals a tall male with a small phallus and small testes.

Klinefelter syndrome

4-y/o presents with new-onset weight loss, polyphagia, and polyuria; PE reveals dehydration but is otherwise normal; glucose is 400 mg/dL.

Insulin-dependent diabetes mellitus (IDDM)

13-y/o obese male presents with a painful limp; frog-leg lateral x-ray shows epiphyseal displacement

Slipped capital femoral epiphysis

10-y/o with h/o sickle cell disease presents in respiratory distress; ↓ hematocrit and ↓ O_2 sat

Acute chest syndrome

2-y/o presents with painless, rectal bleeding; radionuclide scan reveals ectopic gastric mucosa proximal to the ileocecal valve.

Meckel diverticulum

2-y/o presents with fevers and ear pulling; TM is erythematous and bulging without a red reflex

Acute otitis media

12-y/o presents with pain and localized swelling in the distal femur; ↑ alkaline phosphatase and x-ray shows a lytic bone lesion with a "sunburst" appearance

Osteosarcoma

1-mo/o infant with no significant medical history is found to have a III/VI harsh holosystolic murmur heard best at the left lower sternal border on routine examination.

Ventricular septal defect

1-d/o female presents with ambiguous genitalia on newborn exam; labs reveal hyponatremia, hyperkalemia, and hypoglycemia; high levels of 17-hydroxyprogesterone

Congenital adrenal hyperplasia

4-y/o presents with bone pain, arthralgia, and lethargy; PE reveals pallor, ecchymoses, and a fever; labs show anemia and thrombocytopenia.

Acute lymphocytic leukemia

4-y/o presents with barky cough, fever, and rhinorrhea; x-ray reveals "steeple sign."

Croup

8-y/o with h/o bowel and bladder dysfunction presents with a tuft of hair in the lower back; scoliosis is noted on PE.

Spina bifida occulta

5-y/o presents with 6 day h/o high fevers; PE reveals conjunctivitis with limbic sparing, adenitis, strawberry tongue, and fissured lips; platelet count is high and hematocrit is low.

Kawasaki disease

6-y/o child presents after episodes of "daydreaming" in class described as "blank stares"; EEG reveals three-per-second spike and wave pattern.

Absence seizure

3-y/o boy presents with recurrent UTIs; VCUG reveals abnormally placed ureteral insertion into the bladder.

Posterior urethral valve

4-y/o presents with periorbital edema on routine exam; UA reveals severe proteinuria and lipid profile shows hyperlipidemia.

Minimal change disease

8-y/o with h/o sickle cell disease presents with ↑ pallor after viral prodrome; reticulocyte count is <1%

Aplastic crisis

15-y/o presents with fevers and exudative pharyngitis; PE reveals generalized lymphadenopathy; blood smear reveals atypical lymphocytes and heterophile antibody test is positive.

Mononucleosis

1-d/o, 30-week premie presents with retractions, nasal flaring, and cyanosis; CXR shows diffuse atelectasis.

Respiratory distress syndrome

2-mo/o infant presents with respiratory distress and episodic periods of cyanosis; PE reveals right ventricular heave and a loud systolic ejection murmur; CXR shows "boot-shaped heart."

Tetralogy of Fallot

10-y/o presents with fevers and a pruritic rash spreading from the trunk to the arms; PE reveals vesicles of varying stages.

Varicella

8-y/o presents with persistent nighttime coughing; audbile wheezes are heard and mother smokes 2 ppd.

Asthma

15-y/o presents with primary amenorrhea; PE reveals widely spaced nipples, webbed-neck, and a crescendo/decrescendo systolic murmur at the RUSB.

Turner syndrome

Cyanotic newborn presents with respiratory distress; right ventricular heave and a loud S_2; CXR reveals cardiomegaly and an "egg-shaped silhouette."

Transposition of the great vessels

1-mo/o first born male presents with projectile nonbilious vomiting; PE reveals a mobile, non-tender, olive-shaped mass in the epigastric area.

Pyloric stenosis

4-y/o presents with arm pain following trauma; history per mom is inconsisent with injury; x-ray reveals a spiral fracture.

Child abuse

12-y/o presents with symptomatic, episodic palpitations during exercise; ECG reveals "delta waves."

Wolff-Parkinson-White syndrome

3-y/o presents with one generalized seizure lasting 1 min; no significant PMH; PE reveals fevers but is otherwise normal.

Simple febrile seizure

2-wk/o presents with bilious emesis; upper GI series reveals an abnormally placed cecum and ligament of Treitz.

Malrotation

6-mo/o presents with cough, rhinorrhea, and fevers in December; CXR shows peribronchial thickening; nasopharyngeal aspirate reveals RSV antigen.

Bronchiolitis

15-y/o athlete experiences sudden cardiac death during a basketball game; pathologic exam reveals a muscular intraventricular septum and significant LVH.

Hypertrophic obstructive cardiomyopathy

8-y/o presents with fever, photophobia, stiff neck, and headache; PE reveals (+) Kernig and Brudzinski signs; LP shows normal glucose and low WBCs.

Viral meningitis

7-y/o presents with a 1-year h/o leaving seat during class, blurting out answers, and interrupting at home; PE and labs are normal.

Attention-deficit hyperactivity disorder (ADHD)

CHAPTER 7

Emergency Medicine

TRAUMA

List the steps involved in the primary survey of a trauma patient:	"ABCDEFG" (should take <30 s), IV/O$_2$/monitor

Airway: assure clear, unobstructed airway; control cervical spine with back-board or cervical collar.

Breathing: assess chest wall motion; auscultate for bilateral symmetric breath sounds.

Circulation: check pulse, assess vitals, two large-bore IVs with 3:1 isotonic fluid resuscitation, note hemorrhages.

Disability: level of consciousness (GCS), papillary examination, movement of extremities.

Exposure: remove clothing from head to toe to unmask injuries; warm with blankets.

Foley: assess need (contraindicated if blood at urethral meatus, high riding prostate on rectal examination).

Gastric tube: assess need for nasogastric (NG) or oral gastric (OG) tube (contraindicated if concern for basilar skull fracture).

Name six situations that preclude patients with C-spine collars from being cleared clinically (without radiographic imaging):

1. Intoxication (or any altered level of consciousness/inability to communicate)
2. Focal neurologic impairments
3. Posterior midline cervical spine tenderness
4. Painful, distracting injury
5. High-risk mechanism (MVA)
6. Neck rotation to 45° with pain

What method is useful in the evaluation of blunt abdominal trauma?	Focused assessment with sonography for trauma "FAST" (evaluates pericardium, perihepatic, perisplenic, and pelvis)

TOXICOLOGY

What substance supplements gastric lavage in the process of GI decontamination?	Activated charcoal (plus sorbitol for catharsis); CI in AMS, bowel obstruction/perforation, acid/alkali ingestion

For each of the following drugs/toxins, describe the clinical picture of overdose and the antidote/treatment:

Ethylene glycol (antifreeze)	Anion gap metabolic acidosis with $\uparrow$ serum$_{osm}$, calcium oxalate crystals in urine cause renal stones. **Treatment/therapy (Tx):** ethanol, fomepizole, dialysis
Mercury	Erethism (insomnia, delirium, $\downarrow$ memory), peripheral neuropathy, skin discoloration **Tx:** dimercaprol, succimer
Acetaminophen	Ax early, then nausea/vomiting, $\uparrow$ liver function tests (LFTs) and prolonged prothrombin time (PT) at 24-48 h, fulminant hepatic failure at 3-5 days **Tx:** N-acetylcysteine (within 8-10 h)
Warfarin	Bleeding ($\uparrow$ PT/INR) **Tx:** fresh frozen plasma (FFP) (acutely), vitamin K
Antimuscarinics, anticholinergics	"Dry as a bone (dry skin), red as a beet (flushed), blind as a bat (mydriasis), mad as a hatter (delirium)"; Anti-SLUDGE **Tx:** physostigmine (acetylcholinesterase inhibitor)
Digoxin	N/V, dysrhythmias, $\uparrow$ K$^+$, color vision changes (yellow-green haze), AMS **Tx:** manage K$^+$, lidocaine, and antidigoxin Fab

Theophylline	Hematemesis, seizures/coma, dysrhythmias, ↓ BP
	Tx: activated charcoal, cardiac monitoring
Arsenic	Fatigue, seizures; Mees lines in fingernails (chronic)
	Tx: dimercaprol, succimer
Methanol	Anion gap metabolic acidosis with ↑ serum$_{osm}$, blindness (distinguishes from ethylene gycol), optic disc hyperemia
	Tx: ethanol, fomepizole, dialysis
Aspirin (salicylates)	Anion gap metabolic acidosis (normal serum$_{osm}$), respiratory alkalosis, tinnitus, garlic odor
	Tx: alkalinization with bicarb, hemodialysis
Cyanide	Lethargy, loss of consciousness (LOC), dysrhythmias, cherry-red skin color, bitter almond odor
	Tx: sodium thiosulfate and amyl nitrite
Tissue plasminogen activator (tPA), streptokinase	Bleeding
	Tx: aminocaproic acid
Isoniazid (INH)	Peripheral neuropathy, confusion
	Tx: pyridoxine (vitamin B$_6$)
Benzodiazepines	Drowsiness, weakness, ataxia
	Tx: flumazenil (caution in patients on chronic benzos, precipitates seizures)
Lead	Ataxia, peripheral neuropathy, microcytic anemia (with basophilic stippling), lead lines on gums
	Tx: CaEDTA, penicillamine, dimercaprol
Tricyclic antidepressants	**"Three C's"**
	1. Cardiac arrhythmias
	2. Convulsions
	3. Coma
	Tx: Sodium bicarbonate (if QRS >100 ms), benzos for seizures, cardiac monitoring
Alkali agents (drain cleaner, dishwasher detergent)	Mucosal burns, dysphagia, drooling
	Tx: milk/water, then nothing by mouth (NPO)

β-blockers	↓ HR, hypotension, confusion, possible hypoglycemia or ↑ K^+ **Tx:** glucagon, Ca^{2+} (stabilize cardiac membranes)
Heparin	Bleeding (↑ [PTT]), thrombocytopenia **Tx:** protamine sulfate
Opioids	Respiratory and CNS depression, miosis, constipation **Tx:** naloxone (Narcan)
Carbon monoxide (CO)	Headache, confusion, dyspnea, cherry-red skin (later) **Tx:** 100% O_2 or hyperbaric O_2 (if pregnant or CNS dysfunction)
Quinidine	V-tach, torsade de pointes, cinchonism **Tx:** Mg^{2+} (IV)
Iron	Erosive gastritis, N/V, lactic acidosis **Tx:** deferoxamine
Organophosphates (anticholinesterases)	**"SLUDGE"** (Salivation, Lacrimation, Urination, Defacation, Gastric Emptying), wheezing, miosis **Tx:** atropine, pralidoxime
Isopropyl alcohol (rubbing alcohol)	Intoxication, ↓ respiratory rate (RR), ketosis, and elevated osmolar gap (no acidosis) **Tx:** CV/respiratory support, dialysis

ENVIRONMENTAL EMERGENCIES

Name the environmental insult associated with each of the following findings:

Osborne (J) wave on ECG	Hypothermia (<35°C [95°F])
Envenomation may cause local, generalized, or anaphylactic reactions	Hymenoptera (eg, bee stings)
Type of burn initially causing painless, dry, white, cracked, and insensate skin	Full-thickness third-degree- and fourth-degree burns

Loss of thermoregulatory mechanisms, causing CNS dysfunction and dry skin	Heat stroke
Extensive deep-tissue injury under normal skin plus cardiac dysrhythmias	Electrical injury (AC → V-fib; DC → asystole)
Type of burn causing red, blistered, edematous, and painful skin	Partial-thickness (1° and 2°) burns
How is percent of body surface area affected by burns calculated?	Rule of nines: 9% (each arm and head/neck), 18% (each side of torso and each leg), 1% (groin)
When to transfer to burn center	Burn involving >20% total body surface area (TBSA); burn >10% in pt <10 years or >50 years; full thickness burn of >5% TBSA; significant burn of face/hands/genitalia/perineum; significant electrical/chemical/inhalation injury
Sign of inhalation injury	Facial burn, singed nasal hairs, carbonaceous sputum, hypoxia
Fluid resuscitation for burn pts	Parkland Formula (>20% TBSA)— 4 cc × wt (kg) × %TBSA

MAKE THE DIAGNOSIS

75-y/o obese man with h/o of smoking and HTN presents with sudden onset severe abdominal pain, dizziness, and hypotension.

Triple A rupture

27-y/o male s/p MVA and left clavicle fracture presents with shortness of breath (SOB) and left-sided chest pain; PE: cyanotic, decreased breath sounds left side, RR 30, HR 110, BP 90/70, increased JVD

Tension pneumothorax (PTX)

35-y/o woman s/p recent right tibial fracture presents with right leg burning and weakness; PE: capillary refill >2 s, tense skin, numbness in toes

Compartment syndrome

23-y/o man presents with hallucinations, chest pain, and diaphoresis; PE: temp 38°C (100.4°F), HR 118, BP 165/95, and dilated pupils

Cocaine OD

75-y/o man with h/o depression presents with hallucinations and dysrythmia; PE: dilated pupils, warm skin, tachycardia, temp 38.8°C (102°F); w/u: ECG with wide QRS complex

Anti-cholinergic OD, tricyclic antidepressants (TCAs)

Debilitated 70-y/o woman presents with delirium on an August afternoon; PE: dry, hot skin, core body temp 40°C (104°F); w/u: Cr 2.2, UA = myoglobinuria

Heat stroke

40-y/o burn victim presents with headache, dizziness, and confusion; PE: ruddy complexion, oriented to person only, PaO_2 85, arterial blood gas (ABG) 7.30, carboxyhemoglobin (COHb) 17%

CO poisoning

32-y/o woman presents with painful, pruritic skin lesion on arm 4 days after insect bite while camping in southeast United States; PE: violin-shaped lesion with necrotic base and central black eschar, temp 38°C (100.4°F)

Brown recluse spider bite

50-y/o man presents with new onset hematuria and headache; PE: BP 200/180, papilledema

Hypertensive emergency

52-y/o alcoholic male presents with stupor and shivering; PE: temp 27.2°C (81°F), HR 50, RR 9, BP 100/80, dilated pupils; w/u: ECG with J wave

Severe hypothermia

45-y/o woman unrestrained driver in high speed MVA presents obtunded; PE: BP 95/80, HR 132; w/u: CXR: first and second rib fractures, widened mediastinum, loss of aortic knob

Traumatic aortic rupture

32-y/o male burn victim presents with blisters over his chest, abdomen, and both arms. What is TBSA burned?

36%

35-y/o tomato farmer presents with drooling, vomiting, wheezing, and uncontrollable sweating for the past hour; PE: BP 100/70, HR 40, RR 6, miotic pupils, garlic breath, moist skin

Organophosphate poisoning

Abbreviations

AA	amino acid	AV	atrioventricular
Ab	antibody	AXR	abdominal x-ray
ABG	arterial blood gas	AZT	azidothymidine
ABX	antibiotics	BAL	British anti-Lewisite
ACE	angiotensin-converting enzyme	bid	twice daily
ACEI	ACE inhibitor	BM	basement membrane
ACh	acetylcholine	BP	blood pressure
ACL	anterior cruciate ligament	BPH	benign prostatic hyperplasia
ACTH	adrenocorticotropic hormone	BPPV	benign paroxysmal positional vertigo
AD	autosomal dominant	BR	bilirubin
ADH	antidiuretic hormone	BUN	blood urea nitrogen
ADHD	attention-deficit hyperactivity disorder	Bx	biopsy
		CA	cancer/carcinoma
ADP	adenosine diphosphate	CAD	coronary artery disease
AFP	alpha-fetoprotein	cAMP	cyclic adenosine monophosphate
Ag	antigen	CBC	complete blood count
AIDS	acquired immunodeficiency syndrome	CCK	cholecystokinin
		CEA	carcinoembryonic antigen
ALL	acute lymphocytic leukemia	CF	cystic fibrosis
ALP	alkaline phosphatase	CFTR	cystic fibrosis transmembrane regulator
ALS	amyotrophic lateral sclerosis		
ALT	alanine transaminase	cGMP	cyclic guanosine monophosphate
AML	acute myelogenous leukemia		
ANA	antinuclear antibody	CHF	congestive heart failure
ANOVA	analysis of variance	CI	contraindication
ANS	autonomic nervous system	CIN	cervical intraepithelial neoplasia
AR	autosomal recessive	CLL	chronic lymphocytic leukemia
ARB	angiotensin receptor blocker	CML	chronic myelogenous leukemia
ARDS	acute respiratory distress syndrome	CMV	cytomegalovirus
		CN	cranial nerve
ASA	aspirin	CNS	central nervous system
ASD	atrial septal defect	CO	cardiac output
ASO	antistreptolysin O	CoA	coenzyme A
AST	aspartate transaminase	COPD	chronic obstructive pulmonary disease
ATP	adenosine triphosphate		
ATPase	adenosine triphosphatase	COX	cyclooxygenase

CP	cerebral palsy	EPS	extrapyramidal symptoms
CPK	creatine phosphokinase	ER	emergency room
Cr	creatinine	ERCP	endoscopic retrograde
CRF	chronic renal failure		cholangiopancreatography
CRP	c-reactive protein	ESR	erythrocyte sedimentation rate
CS	ceasarean section	ESRD	end-stage renal disease
CSF	cerebrospinal fluid	ESV	end-systolic volume
CT	computed tomography	EtOH	ethanol
CV	cardiovascular	FAs	fatty acids
CVA	cerebrovascular accident *or*	FAP	familial adenomatous polyposis
	costovertebral angle	FFP	fresh frozen plasma
CXR	chest x-ray	FH	family history
d	day(s)	FN	false negatives
D *or* DA	dopamine	FOBT	fecal occult blood test
DAG	diacylglycerol	FP	false positives
DES	diethylstilbestrol	FSH	follicle stimulating hormone
DHT	dihydrotestosterone	FTA-ABS	fluorescent treponemal
DI	diabetes insipidus		antibody—absorption test
DIC	disseminated intravascular	FUO	fever of unknown origin
	coagulation	Fx	fracture
DIP	distal interphalangeal joint	G6PD	glucose-6-phosphate
DKA	diabetic ketoacidosis		dehydrogenase
DM	diabetes mellitus	GABA	γ-aminobutyric acid
DNA	deoxyribonucleic acid	GBM	glomerular BM
DNI	do not intubate	GCT	germ cell tumor
DNR	do not resuscitate	GERD	gastroesophageal reflux disease
d/o	disorder	GFR	glomerular filtration rate
DOE	dyspnea on exertion	GGT	γ-glutamyl transpeptidase
DRE	digital rectal examination	GH	growth hormone
ds	double stranded	GI	gastrointestinal
DSM	*Diagnostic and Statistical*	GN	glomerulonephritis
	Manual of Mental Disorders	GnRH	gonadotropin-releasing
DTP	diphtheria-tetanus-pertussis		hormone
DTR	deep tendon reflex	GTP	guanosine triphosphate
DTs	delirium tremens	GU	genitourinary
DVT	deep venous thrombosis	h	hour(s)
dx	diagnosis *or* diagnose	HA	headache
dz	disease	Hb	hemoglobin
E	epinephrine	HBV	hepatitis B virus
EBV	Epstein-Barr virus	hCG	human chorionic gonadotropin
ECG	electrocardiogram	HDL	high-density lipoprotein
ECT	electroconvulsive therapy	HHV	human herpesvirus
EDV	end-diastolic volume	HIV	human immunodeficiency
EEG	electroencephalogram		virus
EGD	esophagogastroduodenoscopy	HMG-CoA	hydroxymethylglutaryl-CoA
ELISA	enzyme-linked immunosorbent	h/o	history of
	assay	HPA	hypothalamic-pituitary axis
EM	electron microscopy	HPV	human papillomavirus
EOM	extraocular muscle	HR	heart rate

HRT	hormone replacement therapy	MCV	mean corpuscular volume
HSM	hepatosplenomegaly	MEN	multiple endocrine neoplasia
HSV	herpes simplex virus	MHC	major histocompatibility complex
HTLV	human T-cell lymphotrophic virus	MI	myocardial infarction
		MLF	medial longitudinal fasciculus
HTN	hypertension	MMR	measles, mumps, rubella
HUS	hemolytic-uremic syndrome	MOA	mechanism of action
Hx	history	MPTP	1-methyl-4-phenyl-1,2,3,
ICP	intracranial pressure		6-tetrahydropyridine
ICU	intensive care unit	MRI	magnetic resonance imaging
IF	intrinsic factor	MS	multiple sclerosis
Ig	immunoglobulin	MTP	metatarsal-phalangeal
IL	interleukin	MTX	methotrexate
IM	intramuscular	MVA	motor vehicle accident
IND	indication(s)	NE	norepinephrine
INH	isoniazid	NGT	nasogastric tube
INR	International normalized ratio	NOS	not otherwise specified
IOP	intraocular pressure	NPV	negative predictive value
IP_3	inositol triphosphate	NSAID	nonsteroidal anti-inflammatory drug
IPV	inactivated polio vaccine		
IUD	intrauterine device	N/V	nausea/vomiting
IUFD	intra-uterine fetal desease	OA	osteoarthritis
IUGR	intrauterine growth retardation	OCP	oral contraceptive pills
IV	intravenous	OGT	orogastric tube
IVC	inferior vena cava	OPV	oral polio vaccine
IVIG	IV immunoglobulin	PAN	polyarteritis nodosa
JVD	jugular venous distension	p-ANCA	perinuclear pattern of antineutrophil cytoplasmic antibodies
L	left		
LAD	left anterior descending		
LBO	large bowel obstruction	PAS	periodic acid-Schiff (stain)
LCA	left coronary artery	PBS	peripheral blood smear
LDH	lactate dehydrogenase	PCL	posterior cruciate ligament
LDL	low-density lipoprotein	PCP	*Pneumocystis carinii* pneumonia *or* phencyclidine hydrochloride
LES	lower esophageal sphincter		
LFT	liver function test	PCR	polymerase chain reaction
LH	luteinizing hormone	PCWP	pulmonary capillary wedge pressure
LLQ	left lower quadrant		
LLSB	left-lower sternal border	PDA	patent ductus arteriosus
LMN	lower motor neuron	PE	physical examination or pulmonary embolism
LMP	last menstrual period		
LOC	loss of consciousness	PFK	phosphofructokinase
LP	lumbar puncture	PFT	pulmonary function tests
LPS	lipopolysaccharide	PG	prostaglandin
LT	leukotriene	PID	pelvic inflammatory disease
LUQ	left upper quadrant	PIH	pregnancy-induced hypertension
LUSB	left-upper sternal border	PKU	phenylketonuria
LV	left ventricle	PML	progressive mutifocal leucoencephalopathy
MAOI	monoamine oxidase inhibitor		
MCL	medial collateral ligament	PMN	polymorphonuclear

PMR	polymyalgia rheumatica	SGPT	serum glutamic pyruvate transaminase
PNH	paroxysmal nocturnal hemoglobinuria	SLE	systemic lupus erythematosus
PNS	peripheral nervous system	SMX	sulfamethoxazole
PO	by mouth	SOB	shortness of breath
PPD	purified protein derivative	ss	single stranded
PPI	proton pump inhibitor	SSPE	subacute sclerosing panencephalitis
PPRF	parapontine reticular formation		
PPV	positive predictive value	SSRI	selective serotonin reuptake inhibitor
prn	as needed		
PSA	prostate-specific antigen	STD	sexually transmitted disease
Pt	patient	SV	stroke volume
PT	prothrombin time	SVT	supraventricular tachycardia
PTCA	percutaneous transluminal coronary angioplasty	Sx	symptom(s)
		$t_{1/2}$	half-life
PTH	parathyroid hormone	T3	triiodothyronine
PTT	partial thromboplastin time	T4	thyroxine
PUD	peptic ulcer disease	TB	tuberculosis
PVD	peripheral vascular disease	TCA	tricyclic antidepressant
Px	prognosis	TG	triglyceride
R	right	TIBC	total iron-binding capacity
RA	right atrium	TM	tympanic membrane
RAA	renin-angiotensin aldosterone	TMP	trimethoprim
RBC	red blood cell	TN	true negatives
RCA	right coronary artery	TNF	tissue necrosis factor
RDS	respiratory distress syndrome	TNM	tumor, node, metastasis
REM	rapid eye movement	TOX	toxicity
RF	rheumatoid factor	TP	true positives
RLQ	right lower quadrant	tPA	tissue plasminogen activator
ROM	range of motion	TPR	total peripheral resistance
RPR	rapid plasma reagin	TRH	thyrotropin-releasing hormone
RR	respiratory rate	TSH	thyroid-stimulating hormone
RSV	respiratory syncytial virus	TSS	toxic shock syndrome
RTA	renal tubular acidosis	TTP	thrombotic thrombocytopenic purpura
RUQ	right upper quadrant		
RV	right ventricle	Tx	treatment/therapy
RVH	right ventricular hypertrophy	TXA	thromboxane
s	second(s)	UA	urinalysis
S1(2, 3, 4)	1st heart sound (2nd, 3rd, 4th)	UGI	upper GI
SA	sino-atrial	UMN	upper motor neuron
SAH	subarachnoid hemorrhage	URI	upper respiratory infection
SBO	small bowel obstruction	UTI	urinary tract infection
SC	subcutaneous *or* sickle cell	US	ultrasound
SD	standard deviation	VDRL	venereal disease research laboratory
SE	side effects		
SEM	standard error of the mean	Vfib	ventricular fibrillation
SES	socioeconomic status	VHL	von Hippel Lindau
SGOT	serum glutamic oxaloacetic transaminase	VLDL	very-low-density lipoprotein
		VMA	vanillylmandelic acid

V/Q	ventilation/perfusion ratio	5-FU	5-fluorouracil
VSD	ventricular septal defect	5-HIAA	5-hydroxyindoleacetic acid
vWF	von Willebrand factor	5-HT	5-hydroxytryptamine
VZV	varicella-zoster virus		(serotonin)
WBC	white blood cell	↑	High *or* increases
WNL	within normal limits	↓	Low *or* decreases
XL	x-linked	→	Leads to *or* causes
XR	x-ray	~	approximately
y/o	year old	⊕	positive
ZE	Zollinger-Ellison	>>>	much greater than
$1°/2°/3°$	primary/secondary/tertiary	<<<	much less than

Index

Lightning Source UK Ltd.
Milton Keynes UK
UKHW021056050419
340503UK00005B/362/P